Notes on Pathology for Small Animal Clinicians

A Veterinary Practitioner Handbook
Series Edited by Neal King BVSC MRCVS

NOTES ON PATHOLOGY FOR SMALL ANIMAL CLINICIANS

D. F. Kelly MA, PhD, BVSc, MRCVS, FRCPath
Professor of Veterinary Pathology
University of Liverpool

V. M. Lucke PhD, BVSc, FRCVS
Senior Lecturer in Veterinary Pathology,
University of Bristol

C. J. Gaskell PhD, BVSc, DVR, MRCVS
Lecturer in Veterinary Medicine,
University of Bristol

WRIGHT·PSG

Bristol   London   Boston
1982

Published by:
John Wright & Sons Ltd, 42–44 Triangle West,
Bristol BS8 1EX, England

John Wright PSG Inc.,
545 Great Road, Littleton, Massachusetts 01460, USA.

British Library Cataloguing in Publication Data
Kelly, D. F.
    Notes on pathology for small animal clinicians
    (A Veterinary practitioner handbook)
    1. Veterinary pathology
    I. Title   II. Lucke, V. M.   III. Gaskell, C. J.
    IV. Series
    636.089'607   SF769

ISBN 0 7236 0657 9

Library of Congress Catalog Card Number: 81-70759

Typeset by
Activity, Salisbury, Wilts
and printed in Great Britain by
John Wright & Sons (Printing) Ltd, at the Stonebridge Press, Bristol BS4 5NU

Preface

This book provides an outline of some practical approaches to the pathology of dogs and cats for veterinary surgeons in small animal practice. There are two separate, but related reasons for writing this book. Present courses in pathology for undergraduate veterinary students necessarily have to emphasize the general principles of cellular and tissue pathology and relatively less time is available for formal teaching in some of the more practical aspects of surgical, clinical and post-mortem pathology. Regrettable though this may be, the trend is welcomed by some and accepted as inevitable by others, who recognize that special training in pathology is more appropriately a postgraduate activity. The second reason is simply that small animal clinicians soon realize the need for a more detailed understanding of pathology than undergraduate courses provide, and the practice of small animal medicine requires a practical familiarity with haematology, clinical and surgical pathology and morbid anatomy.

The small animal practitioner utilizes clinical chemistry and haematology widely as aids to diagnosis and clinical management. Chapter 1 outlines the procedures in these areas that are currently useful to the small animal clinician: it deals with the functional rationale of the tests and emphasizes the diagnostic uses and limitations of methods presently in use. Small animal surgeons increasingly need to work closely with practising veterinary pathologists to provide histological diagnoses, to confirm the adequacy of surgical excision and to provide an objective basis for prognosis. Surgical pathology is particularly important in the approach to skin and mammary tumours. Chapters 2 and 3 deal with these important areas of practical pathology, emphasizing the clinical features of cutaneous and mammary neoplasms and outlining the clinical significance of the histological terminology used in their diagnosis.

Small animal clinicians may also be required to carry out post-mortem examinations. For useful information to be derived from this, and for the individual practitioner to build a base of firm experience, it is advisable to follow a systematic approach to the small animal post-mortem examination (Chapter 4). Assessment of the possible clinical significance of changes found at necropsy requires, first, a knowledge of common agonal and post-mortem changes from which putative ante-mortem lesions have to be distinguished (Chapter 5). Of equal importance in the necropsy is an appreciation of the existence of clinically silent or trivial lesions which may be associated with ageing and which are of no functional significance. Chapter 6 deals with the macroscopic lesions found commonly as incidental post-mortem findings in dogs and cats.

The emphasis throughout these chapters is on those aspects of pathology that are relevant to small animal practice: the result is intended to be a textbook neither of clinical pathology nor of diagnostic morbid anatomy, but is an attempt to provide insight into the contribution that these areas of pathology can make to clinical diagnosis, patient management and understanding of disease processes. The choice of a clinician to write Chapter 1 is a deliberate one consistent with the approach outlined above: the author has experience of small animal medical practice in which clinical chemistry and haematology are used extensively and is therefore involved in critical assessment of the contributions that these laboratory aids make to clinical veterinary medicine.

The authors have drawn upon their experiences in clinical and pathology practice in university veterinary schools and gratefully acknowledge the contributions made by their colleagues to the ideas, practices and observations that are presented in this book. The authors alone are responsible for any error of fact or interpretation and would welcome correction or discussion on contentious points. We have chosen to be dogmatic and to minimize discussion in the latter areas where we believe this to be consistent with the clinical orientation and the note form of the book.

We are grateful to J. Conibear, C. C. Jeal, Paula Jenkins and Jo Minns for the illustrations, and to Pam Denning and Valerie Gardiner for secretarial assistance.

D.F.K.
V.M.L.
C.J.G.

Contents

Chapter 1

Clinical Pathology and Haematology in Small Animal Medicine

This chapter attempts to provide a logical approach to the use of laboratory tests in the investigation of the major presenting clinical signs encountered in small animal practice. The emphasis placed on laboratory data, however, in no way suggests that they should replace or even precede the thorough taking of a history and clinical examination, both of which are always cheaper and frequently more rewarding. The apparent objectivity of laboratory results is always appealing but the over-reliance on such information, particularly when based on a single result, is unwise, and whenever such information is at variance with the clinical impression, the laboratory tests should be repeated.

The laboratory tests discussed are, to a great extent, those which are readily available, either within a practice or from a commercial laboratory, and thus the text is not a complete guide to laboratory techniques. Neither does the chapter attempt to cover every possible condition that might be associated with a particular clinical sign. To do so would require a medical textbook, which this is not. In a further attempt to be succinct, some generalizations have been made with which some might not agree or with which individual cases might not fit.

DIARRHOEA AND VOMITING

Laboratory tests are probably of most use in the investigation of chronic, as opposed to acute, diarrhoea and vomiting. In the majority of acute cases, such as intestinal obstruction or haemorrhagic gastroenteritis (HGE), their use is often not justified and other diagnostic aids, such as radiography, may be more rewarding. Some exceptions to this generalization are considered below, followed by an approach to cases of chronic vomiting and diarrhoea.

Acute

Acute vomiting and diarrhoea may be part of a wider clinical syndrome where laboratory data may be of benefit. Examples include the use of haematology in pyometritis (p. 8) and amylase and lipase estimations in acute pancreatitis (p. 12). Vomiting may be a major sign in acute renal failure where blood urea, creatinine and potassium levels are elevated; urine production is minimal (oliguria), what is produced being concentrated and containing red blood cells (RBCs), tubular casts and cellular debris. Where renal failure follows a period of compensated chronic renal disease the history may include polydipsia (*see* p. 5). Viral infections, e.g. parvoviruses of dogs (CPV) and cats (FIE); coronavirus of dogs and rotavirus of cats, also cause acute vomiting and diarrhoea. Their identification may be carried out by specialist laboratories but the confirmation of the diagnosis is often retrospective.

Chronic

In chronic diarrhoea, some diagnostic information such as the type of diarrhoea, i.e. whether originating from the large or small bowel, may be obtained from the appearance of the faeces. The presence of mucus in (or occasionally passed separately from) the faeces and fresh blood streaked in the faecal motion are indicative of large bowel disease, e.g. colitis. There are no confirmatory laboratory tests for colitis, and even proctoscopy and biopsy may be disappointing as mucosal changes may be minimal. Dark tarry faeces (melaena) are evidence of haemorrhage in the upper gastro-intestinal tract (e.g. gastric or small bowel ulceration, benign or neoplastic) and the subsequent partial digestion of the blood. Acute and profound haemorrhage is seen with haemorrhagic gastroenteritis (HGE) in dogs and is also reported with canine parvovirus infection. Specific tests for blood in faeces have the considerable disadvantage of reacting with normal dietary haemoglobin. The need, therefore, to feed a haemoglobin-free diet prior to assessment (for about 3 days) makes such tests largely impracticable. The consistent finding of melaena is an indication for contrast radiography of the bowel or exploratory laparotomy.

Pale, fatty and voluminous faeces are characteristic of malabsorption due to exocrine pancreatic insufficiency (EPI), the presence of which may be confirmed by laboratory tests.

In many cases of chronic diarrhoea, however, the gross appearance of the faeces is unremarkable and further differentiation relies on laboratory data.

Faecal examination

Muscle fibres and fat: The demonstration of undigested muscle fibres and fat in faecal smears suggests malabsorption but is less specific than other tests for, say, pancreatic insufficiency.

Parasites: The examination of samples for evidence of parasitic and coccidial infection is relevant in the routine screening of cases with chronic diarrhoea, though their presence may be incidental and their significance can often only be assessed from the response to treatment.

Bacteriology: The value of bacterial culture of faeces in cases of chronic diarrhoea is strictly limited. While bacterial overgrowth may exacerbate diarrhoea, particularly where maldigestion and malabsorption is occurring, the underlying problem is not usually bacterial. The significance of the presence of salmonella and haemolytic *Escherichia coli* may be more difficult to interpret, but these too are often incidental to some underlying primary disease. In young animals, however, bacterial culture and anti-biotic sensitivity testing may be more relevant.

Faecal trypsin: Faecal trypsin levels are extremely variable in normal dogs; at least three samples should be tested and only consistently negative or low levels of trypsin activity be accepted as diagnostic of EPI. A more specific test, based on the oral administration of a synthetic substrate for a pancreatic enzyme (chymotrypsin) and the subsequent measurement of its breakdown product (PABA) in blood or urine, has been described and may be helpful in some cases (Appendix 1.1). The clinical observation that some dogs with normal or only marginally low levels of faecal trypsin show some response to therapy with pancreatic enzymes is difficult to explain, but should not be taken as confirmation of typical EPI.

Absorption tests

In cases of malabsorption due, for example, to lymphosarcoma of the bowel, villous atrophy, eosinophilic gastroenteritis or lymphangiectasia, faecal examination is often unrewarding and more sophisticated tests are necessary.

Xylose absorption: A severe loss of absorptive capacity can lead to a reduction in xylose uptake by the small bowel as assessed by blood levels following oral administration of this sugar (Appendix 1.2). Glucose, which is cheaper but less specific, may be used instead. However, the results of xylose absorption must be interpreted with caution as bowel lesions and clinical (i.e. dietary) malabsorption may be present with apparently normal absorption of xylose or glucose. Slow gastric emptying due, for example, to prior feeding, will lead to delayed xylose absorption and even where reduced absorption is due to small intestinal disease, confirmation and precise definition of the diagnosis will require bowel biopsy.

Other absorption tests: The measurement of fat absorption in the diagnosis of pancreatic insufficiency has been described but is time-consuming and unpleasant. Similarly digestion and absorption of a disaccharide, e.g. lactose, has been measured but is rarely used in practice.

Haematology

Eosinophilic gastroenteritis, usually associated with a less severe malabsorption syndrome, is characterized by a circulating eosinophilia
($>1000/\mu l$), though the degree of eosinophilia may vary between samples.

Haematological examination is not helpful in differentiating the other
causes of malabsorption; lymphosarcoma of the bowel is rarely, if ever,
truly leukaemic and cases may indeed show a lymphopenia. Rarely, malabsorption may lead to a severe reduction in folic acid and vitamin B_6
(pyridoxine) uptake and anaemia results.

Blood biochemistry

Protein: In the rare cases of lymphangiectasia, and in some cases of
lymphosarcoma of the bowel, malabsorption may be accompanied by
protein loss into the bowel lumen. In such protein-losing enteropathy
there is a reduction in plasma albumin and globulin and as a result of the
reduced osmotic pressure of plasma, subcutaneous oedema and ascites
may develop.

Intestinal biopsy

In the majority of cases confirmation of the presence and cause of malabsorption requires intestinal biopsy (Appendix 1.3). However, with the
present poor understanding of the aetiology and pathogenesis of the
recognized causes of malabsorption such a precise diagnosis may not
radically alter the clinical management of the case.

Chronic diarrhoea of dietary origin, e.g. milk intolerance in the cat, and
the so-called 'functional diarrhoeas' seen in large dogs, are commonly
encountered in practice but laboratory data are of little diagnostic value.
Chronic vomiting or regurgitation due to gastric or oesophageal disease,
e.g. gastric carcinoma, megoesophagus and cases of chronic diarrhoea and
vomiting due to partial obstruction of the bowel, do not lend themselves
to laboratory investigation, other techniques, e.g. radiography or
exploratory surgery, being more appropriate. Exceptions are the demonstration of changed blood (melaena) in the faeces of cases with upper
alimentary tract bleeding, and the demonstration of indican in the urine
in the presence of bowel obstruction. Both tests are, however, of limited
value. The interpretation of faecal blood has been discussed above (p. 2)
and the presence of indican, the product of bacterial breakdown of
tryptophan, is by no means specific for obstruction.

Other conditions that may show chronic vomiting and diarrhoea and in
which laboratory tests are helpful include chronic renal failure (p. 5),
liver disease, either chronic (p. 11) or obstructive (p. 13), hypoadrenocorticalism (Addison's disease) (p. 20) and the ketoacidosis of diabetes
mellitus (p. 5).

POLYDIPSIA AND POLYURIA

The conditions most commonly associated with these two signs in the dog are:

    Chronic renal failure of any cause.
    Pyometritis.
    Diabetes mellitus.
    Hyperadrenocorticalism (Cushing's syndrome).
    Diabetes insipidus.
    Liver failure.

In the cat, chronic renal failure is by far the commonest cause of poly-dipsia recognized. A normal dog drinks about 50 ml/kg body weight per day, while a cat drinks between 20 and 100 ml per day; in both species the level will be influenced greatly by the moisture content and formulation of the food. An initial history should attempt to eliminate environmental (e.g. diet, temperature), iatrogenic (e.g. corticosterioid or diuretic therapy) or other (e.g. oestrus) causes for increased thirst and some estimate of the degree of polydipsia should be made. The polydipsia noticed by the owner is frequently secondary to polyuria. In the majority of cases of polydipsia laboratory tests are important diagnostically though the presence of other clinical signs may suggest one diagnosis. In pyometritis, laboratory data may be less crucial and other diagnostic aids, e.g. radiography, may be more helpful. In the investigation of polydipsic animals, it should be remembered that conditions may often co-exist, e.g. renal failure and pyometritis, renal failure and diabetes mellitus.

Urinanalysis

Urinanalysis should be the first laboratory test employed.

Glycosuria

The presence of definite glycosuria ($>0\cdot5$ per cent) is usually indicative of diabetes mellitus. Intensive intravenous glucose fluid therapy may cause transient glycosuria, and occasional cases of hyperadrenocorticalism and acute renal tubular disease may also be associated with mild glycosuria. In Fanconi's syndrome — a rarely recognized renal tubular defect resulting in reduced tubular resorption of glucose — glycosuria also occurs but in the presence of normal plasma levels of glucose.

The use of Clinitest tablets is generally considered a more reliable guide to urine glucose levels than Clinistix paper strips.* Confirmation of diabetes mellitus and the elimination of other causes of glycosuria may be made by the demonstration of hyperglycaemia ($>6\cdot00$ mmol/1). Ketones

---

*Clinitest and Clinistix, Ames Co., Division of Miles Laboratories Ltd, Slough, Berks.

are not normally found in urine but may be present in diabetes mellitus and are, as a reflection of ketoacidosis, important clinically; ketonuria is not present in any other common condition of the dog or cat.

Proteinuria

The presence of proteinuria is often taken as an indication of renal disease, particularly chronic renal failure, but this is too simplistic a view. Protein is a normal, though minor, constituent of urine and, especially in the cat, may be readily appreciated in concentrated urine. In chronic renal failure, protein is lost from the kidneys, but while urine concentrations of protein may be elevated (30–300 mg/dl) they may also vary considerably and, in the dilute urine produced, be only of the order of 10–20 mg/dl. In addition, care must be taken in the interpretation of urine test sticks as the measurement of protein levels may be unreliable if urine pH varies appreciably from the normal range, and other tests, such as the sulphosalicylic acid test, are to be preferred. Where the presence of protein in urine suggests chronic renal failure, the measurement of blood urea is indicated. The proteinuria associated with glomerulonephritis in both dog and cat, and in the dog with amyloidosis, is much greater than in chronic renal failure, in the order of grammes, rather than milligrammes per decilitre. Glomerulonephritis may, as one of the causes of chronic renal failure, be associated with polydipsia and polyuria, but in the early stages of the disease these signs are usually absent. Proteinuria will also be present in any urinary tract infection or haemorrhage, together with other evidence of the primary disease, i.e. white and red blood cells, bacteria.

Urine specific gravity

Though variable in the normal animal, it may be of diagnostic help and some guidelines are given below:

Chronic renal failure	1008–1012
Diabetes mellitus	Usually >1040
Hyperadrenocorticalism	1006–1020, though can concentrate further
Diabetes insipidus	<1008
Pyometritis, liver failure	Variable
Normal Dog	1015–1045
Cat	1020–1050

Values for urine osmolarity give essentially the same information as those for specific gravity.

Urine pH

Urine pH is classically acidic (5·8–6·5) in decompensated chronic renal failure and ketoacidotic diabetes mellitus, though this may be confused by the presence of intercurrent urinary tract infection. Such infection is not uncommon in diabetes mellitus and may occur in hyperadrenocorticalism. Urine samples left at room temperature for 12-24 hours will become progressively more alkaline because of the breakdown of urea.

Urine sediment

The finding of a few red and white blood cells in urine sediment may be normal, though the presence of large numbers, and a positive test for blood in the urine, is usually indicative of urinary infection. Large numbers of casts, either hyaline or cellular, in urine sediment suggest active tubular disease. Crystal deposits are not usually of clinical significance, with the exception of ammonium urate crystals which may be associated with liver failure, and heavy calcium oxalate deposits seen in ethylene glycol (antifreeze) poisoning. Urate deposits, however, may be normal in Dalmatian dogs. A more extensive guide to the interpretation of urine sediments may be found in other texts (e.g. Bush, 1975).

Blood biochemistry

Urea

Of the blood biochemical tests, blood urea is the simplest indicator of renal function and given the frequency of chronic renal failure as a primary or complicating factor in polydipsia, it should be measured routinely in such cases. The degree of elevation of blood urea is not always related to the severity of clinical signs but in general terms signs of chronic renal failure are often slight with a blood urea level below 20 mmol/l: where the level has risen to 60 mmol/l and above, the prognosis is very poor in the absence of any reversible, post-renal (i.e. obstructive) component. Elevation in blood urea of up to about 20 mmol/l may in some circumstances be due to pre-renal factors (e.g. dehydration, cardiac insufficiency).

In hyperadrenocorticalism blood urea is usually normal; it may be raised in ketoacidotic diabetes mellitus due to dehydration and may be normal or raised in pyometritis. Blood urea is sometimes low in cases of diabetes insipidus, presumably due to reduced tubular resorption of urea, and is invariably low ($<2\cdot5$ mmol/l) in dogs with hepatic failure or portasystemic shunting where urea production in the liver is reduced; low blood urea levels are here a crude assessment of liver function (*see* p. 11).

Creatinine

Plasma creatinine levels are also raised in renal failure but smaller amounts are present and measurement may require more plasma. Creatinine is of greater value than urea in monitoring renal function where protein metabolite production is being controlled by diet as part of the management of chronic renal failure.

Inorganic phosphorus

Plasma inorganic phosphorus may also rise in chronic renal failure; it should be remembered that levels are higher in normal young animals than in adults by a factor of about 1·5.

Others

Plasma calcium is sometimes low, and potassium may be elevated in the terminal stages of renal decompensation. The biochemical demonstration of reduced renal function gives no indication of the underlying renal pathology, though where this is due to glomerulonephritis or, in the dog, amyloidosis, plasma albumin levels will be reduced (<25 g/l) owing to protein loss in the urine.

Of the other commonly employed biochemical parameters few are important diagnostically in cases of polydipsia, though some may be abnormal. The fatty infiltration of the liver seen in both diabetes mellitus and hyperadrenocorticalism frequently leads to elevated serum (or plasma) levels of the enzymes alkaline phosphatase (SAP) and glutamate pyruvate transaminase (SGPT/ALT) more particularly the former (up to 250 i.u./l). Plasma cholesterol levels may also be elevated in these two conditions. These changes are reversible with successful treatment. SGPT and SAP, together with plasma protein levels, may also be abnormal in liver failure; this situation is considered in detail under ascites (p. 9).

Haematology

Haematology is of value in the diagnosis of pyometritis and hyperadrenocorticalism. A marked neutrophilia (often >30·0 x 10^3/μl) and the presence of immature band forms (shift to the left) are compatible with a diagnosis of pyometritis; this elevation may be visible grossly as a deep (3 mm+) buffy coat on a capillary haematocrit (normal buffy coat approximately 1 mm deep). In hyperadrenocorticalism lymphopenia and absolute eosinopenia are often present, though the presence of a neutrophilia often makes the total WBC count normal or slightly elevated. A neutrophilia may also be present in diabetes mellitus due to intercurrent infection, e.g. cystitis. Animals in chronic renal failure often have a non-regenerative anaemia resulting from a reduced lifespan of the red cells and lowered erythropoietin production by the damaged kidney.

Plasma cortisol

Demonstration of a lymphopenia and eosinopenia in the presence of a normal blood urea and typical clinical signs is usually sufficient basis for a diagnosis of hyperadrenocorticalism, though the haematological findings do not allow differentiation between the various causes of the syndrome (idiopathic adrenocortical hyperplasia, adrenocortical hyperplasia associated with a pituitary tumour and adrenocortical tumour). Confirmation of the diagnosis may be achieved by measuring plasma cortisol levels.

A resting cortisol level alone is often of little value as normal and abnormal ranges overlap considerably, but a level of >550 nmol/l following ACTH stimulation (0·125–0·250 mg of ACTH* i.m., sample taken ½ or 2 hours later) may be considered diagnostic of hyperadrenocorticalism. The measurement of plasma cortisol following dexamethasone suppression has been described for the differentiation of adrenocortical hyperplasia and adrenocortical tumour but is of limited practical value as results may be equivocal and adrenal tumours are, in any case, an uncommon cause of hyperadrenocorticalism. In iatrogenic Cushing's syndrome, i.e. that caused by long-term steroid treatment, both resting and 'stimulated' cortisol levels are low unless cortisol itself has been used in therapy.

Urine concentration tests

The occurrence of a low urine specific gravity in the absence of any other abnormality indicates by exclusion the presence of diabetes insipidus. Where this is caused by a failure of antidiuretic hormone (ADH) to reach the renal tubules, the diagnosis may be confirmed first by an inability of the animal to concentrate urine following water restriction (water restriction test, Appendix 1.4), and secondly by the urine concentration (to specific gravity >1020) which follows the administration of exogenous ADH.

In the past, natural vasopressin tannate† (in oil) was given as exogenous ADH but this is no longer available and a synthetic analog‡ is now used (dose 1·3 µg for animals up to 15 kg body weight; 2·7 µg above 15 kg body weight). An animal that fails to concentrate urine following either water restriction or ADH administration is said to have nephrogenic diabetes insipidus (in which the renal tubules seem relatively less responsive to the effects of ADH). In psychogenic, or compulsive polydipsia, water restriction should lead to urine concentration although in long-standing cases the ability to concentrate may be temporarily reduced and more gradual restriction needed.

ASCITES

Though strictly referring to serous fluids, the accumulation of appreciable amounts of any fluid in the peritoneal cavity is frequently referred to as

---

*Synacthen, Ciba Labs, Horsham, Sussex.
†Pitressin, Parke, Davis & Co., Pontypool, Gwent.
‡Desmopressin (DDAVP), Ferring Pharmaceuticals Ltd, Twickenham, Middlesex.

ascites. This is appreciated clinically as abdominal distension, often with a palpable fluid wave, and radiographically as a loss of abdominal soft-tissue contrast. Differentiation of the causes is based initially on an examination of the fluid in the light of the clinical signs (for the technique of para-centesis, *see* Appendix 1.5). Such fluids may be classified as blood, chyle, transudates or exudates: of these transudates and blood are most commonly encountered.

Blood

The presence of blood in the abdominal cavity (which does not clot, in contrast to blood withdrawn from an organ such as the spleen) suggests either trauma to a blood vessel or parenchymatous organ (which may be surgical), abdominal neoplasia (typically splenic haemangiosarcoma) or less commonly a bleeding disorder (e.g. Warfarin poisoning, thrombocytopenia). In acute abdominal haemorrhage (i.e. less than 12 hours) the loss of circulating red cells will not be reflected in the PCV or haemoglobin con-centration as blood volume has not been replenished, and thus haematol-ogy is of little clinical use in assessing the degree of anaemia. The assess-ment of clotting function in such cases is dealt with elsewhere (persistent haemorrhage, p. 19). Management of such cases (fluid replacement, blood transfusion, exploratory laparotomy) is based primarily on a clinical assessment of the animal rather than on laboratory results.

Chyle

The finding of chyle in the peritoneal cavity is rare; such fluid is thick and milky and contains large numbers of lymphocytes and amounts of fat. It results from traumatic or neoplastic damage to major lymphatics.

Transudate

The differentiation of the cause of ascites becomes more complex when the fluid is a transudate (i.e. a low protein, non-inflammatory, watery fluid) or a modified transudate (i.e. a similar fluid with some protein, but <30 g/l and often bloodstained).

Peritoneal transudates may be associated with either hypoproteinaemia, portal vein hypertension, or, in the case of chronic liver disease, a combination of the two.

Hypoproteinaemia

True unmodified transudates are most frequently associated with a lowering of the osmotic pressure of plasma due to a reduction in protein concentration (hypoproteinaemia). The hypoproteinaemia may be related to loss of protein from either the small intestine or kidneys or to a reduced production by the liver. It is frequently accompanied by dependent subcutaneous oedema, especially in the cat. Rarely is it due to insufficient dietary protein. Protein-losing nephropathies (glomerulonephritis and amyloidosis in the dog) may be demonstrated by the presence of large amounts ($>$1 g/dl) of protein in the urine and a marked reduction (to $<$25 g/l) in plasma albumin. The underlying cause may be defined specifically by kidney biopsy. In glomerulonephritis blood urea levels are often normal though such cases may, over a period of months, develop chronic renal failure. Plasma globulin levels may be elevated in glomerulonephritis as may cholesterol levels. Protein-losing enteropathies (e.g. lymphosarcoma of the intestine, lymphangiectasia) are invariably associated with diarrhoea and more typically show a reduction in both plasma albumin and globulin. Impaired intestinal absorption may be demonstrated by xylose absorption test (*see* Diarrhoea, p. 3) but again biopsy of the organ is necessary for a specific diagnosis (Appendix 1.3.)

Hypoproteinaemia associated with chronic liver failure may also lead to the formation of a peritoneal transudate, though the formation of such a transudate is frequently due to a combination of reduced plasma protein levels and portal hypertension secondary to liver fibrosis. The transudate so formed is often 'modified'.

Portal hypertension

Portal hypertension is caused in the majority of cases by either chronic hepatic disease with fibrosis, right-sided congestive heart failure or neoplasia.

Laboratory substantiation of a diagnosis of hepatic fibrosis following chronic liver disease relies on the demonstration of reduced function. Such cases may not show jaundice. A crude, but useful, assessment may be made from the low levels of plasma albumin ($<$25 g/l) and urea ($<$2·5 mmol/l) but the injection of BSP and the measurement of the amount remaining in the plasma at 30 min (BSP retention test, *see* Appendix 1.6) is a better assessment of liver function and if repeated allows comparisons to be made over a period of time. A normal dog retains less than 5 per cent of injected BSP at 30 minutes and long term prognosis is guarded when this rises to $>$20 per cent, though in the short term such animals may do well on treatment, particularly dietary management. Experience with BSP in the cat is limited, but the principle of the technique is the same.

Liver enzyme levels reflect liver pathology but should not be considered as function tests. In chronic liver failure, due for example to a chronic hepatitis, SGPT may be only slightly raised (approx. 50 i.u./l) and SAP just moderately so (100–200 i.u./l). Blood ammonia levels, either resting or following alimentary loading with ammonia (ammonia tolerance test), are often raised in chronic liver disease particularly where this is associated with congenital or acquired portasystemic shunting of blood. The measurement of ammonia must be made quickly, within 20 min of sampling.

The other major cause of a modified transudate ascites is right-sided congestive heart failure where the pathogenesis is similarly portal hypertension. A definitive diagnosis of congestive heart failure relies on clinical, radiographic and electrocardiographic (ECG) examination of the cardiovascular system.

Ascites due to a modified transudate may also occur when an abdominal neoplasm obstructs venous or lymphatic flow. Most commonly these involve the liver, either primarily or secondarily, and may lead to elevations in liver enzyme levels. Cytological examination of ascitic fluid for neoplastic cells requires considerable skill and is often disappointing in the hands of an inexperienced cytologist. Confirmation of a diagnosis with or without biochemical evidence of specific organ dysfunction requires exploratory laparotomy.

Exudate

The finding of large amounts of inflammatory exudate sufficient to cause abdominal distension is uncommon except in feline infectious peritonitis (FIP) when the fluid is thick, straw-coloured, high in protein and fibrin, and clots on standing. In cases of FIP there is a hypergammaglobulinaemia (>50 g/l) and 50 per cent of cases have a non-regenerative anaemia. Examination for feline leukaemia virus (FeLV) may be appropriate in a colony animal due to the epidemiological association between this agent and FIP. There is at present no *in vivo* confirmatory test for FIP, though coronavirus serology is offered diagnostically in some countries.

Serosanguineous exudates may indicate a chemical peritonitis such as that caused by leakage of bile, urine or pancreatic enzyme. The volume of resultant 'ascitic' fluid in such cases is frequently small and paracentesis may be unrewarding or result in only a small sample being obtained. The finding of bilirubin or urea/creatinine in greater concentration in the ascitic fluid than in plasma will confirm the diagnosis and in such cases blood biochemistry will show evidence of hepatic or renal failure. Pancreatitis and the associated peritonitis is typically associated with a rise in plasma amylase. Doubts concerning the specificity and persistence of elevated values, however, make their interpretation difficult and only a massive rise (>2000 i.u./l amylase) can be considered positively diagnostic and a normal value may not exclude the diagnosis. Purulent exudates, with large numbers of neutrophils and macrophages present in the fluid, may form following penetrating wounds, abdominal surgery, intestinal perforation or the rupture of a pyometra or other infectious focus, but are frequently localized by mesentery. They are associated, as is any case of inflammatory peritonitis, chemical or infectious, with a circulating neutrophilia.

JAUNDICE

The presence of clinical jaundice does not necessarily imply that there is primary liver disease, nor is severe liver disease always associated with jaundice. Laboratory investigation is aimed at defining the cause of the jaundice as pre-hepatic (haemolytic), hepatic or post-hepatic (obstructive).

Bilirubin

The type of jaundice can usually be assessed by separating the total bilirubin concentration in the blood, which in itself gives merely an objective measure of the clinically apparent jaundice, into unconjugated (indirect reacting) and conjugated (direct reacting) forms (van den Bergh test). In pre-hepatic jaundice the unconjugated form of bilirubin predominates (>90 per cent of total) as bilirubin produced by RBC breakdown exceeds the 'conjugating' capacity of the normal liver. In post-hepatic jaundice the conjugated bilirubin formed in the liver is not excreted by the biliary system and refluxes into the blood, typically forming the bulk (>80 per cent) of the total blood bilirubin level. Hepatic jaundice, due to hepatocellular damage, is characterized by a variable mixture of unconjugated and conjugated bilirubin. However, a distinction between hepatic and post-hepatic jaundice may not be possible on bilirubin results alone.

Liver enzymes

Liver enzyme levels are also helpful in defining the type of jaundice. SAP is typically raised in post-hepatic, or obstructive, biliary disease though levels may also be raised when there is intrahepatic biliary stasis due to liver cell necrosis and fibrosis; elevations in SGPT indicate hepatocyte damage and are thus most marked in hepatic jaundice. As expected, both SAP and SGPT are normal in pre-hepatic jaundice, unless the anaemia is profound (*see below*).

Several factors, however, must be remembered in interpreting levels of SAP.

1. SAP is produced by various body tissues; increased production, leading to raised serum levels, is seen in the absence of liver or biliary disease, e.g. in young animals (during skeletal growth, i.e. <9 months of age), in bone disease and, rarely, in certain forms of neoplastic disease.

2. Intrahepatic biliary stasis caused by fatty infiltration in diabetes mellitus or hyperadrenocorticalism, will lead to elevation in SAP (of the order of 2–300 i.u./l) in the absence of primary liver or biliary disease.

3. The cat, unlike the dog, can excrete SAP via the kidneys and thus elevation of serum levels of AP is a less useful indication of biliary stasis in this species.

SGPT, being liver-derived, is generally easier to interpret, though slight elevation (up to 50 i.u./l) may be difficult to explain clinically and some increase may be seen in profound anaemia or congestive heart failure due to centrilobular hypoxia and necrosis. Serum glutamic oxaloacetate trans-aminase (SGOT) is of little value as an indicator of liver damage in dogs and cats as the enzyme is produced by a number of other body tissues; the same is true for lactate dehydrogenase (LDH) (unless isoenzyme studies are carried out). Enzymes such as gamma-glutamyl-transpeptidase (γGT) and sorbitol dehydrogenase (SDH), often offered in medical blood bio-chemistry profiles, may be of value clinically in the dog and cat but experience is limited.

Urinanalysis

The presence of bile pigments in urine — bilirubinuria — occurs readily in the dog and cat with increased levels of conjugated bilirubin in the blood (unconjugated bilirubin is too large to pass through the glomerulus, as it is bound to plasma albumin). However, up to 60 per cent of normal dogs and 5 per cent of cats will show a weak positive reaction to tests for bilirubin in urine. Strongly positive reactions are a useful indicator of jaundice and are seen with obstructive biliary tract disease. Urobilinogen, formed from the breakdown of conjugated bilirubin in the bowel, is present in normal urine; changes in urine concentration are used to differentiate between types of jaundice and man but are of little routine value in the dog and cat.

Haematology

Pre-hepatic jaundice, being haemolytic in origin, is associated with an anaemia which is invariably regenerative in type. Examination of a blood smear stained with Giemsa's stain (for blood parasites, e.g. *Haemobartonella felis*), the use of techniques to demonstrate the presence of autoimmune disease (Coombs antiglobulin test, Papain test, anti-nuclear antibody test) or, in cats, examination of blood for FeLV, may indicate the cause of the haemolysis (*see also* p. 17).

Haematological changes in hepatic jaundice are variable but usually consist of a moderate neutrophilia which is not helpful diagnostically. Early cases of canine hepatitis (ICH) may show a neutropenia. Other appropriate laboratory tests in cases of hepatic jaundice include the microscopic examination of fresh urine under dark ground illumination for the presence of leptospiral organisms, more subtle assessments of liver function, e.g. BSP retention (*see* Ascites, p. 11), paired serum samples (acute and convalescent) for measurement of antibody response to the adenovirus of ICH, and liver biopsy.

The demonstration of pure post-hepatic jaundice is usually an indication for exploratory laparotomy since most cases in dogs and cats are associated with abdominal neoplasia.

DYSPNOEA AND TACHYPNOEA

In many cases of dyspnoea, or difficulty in breathing, laboratory data have little place in the diagnosis. Exceptions include cases of tachypnoea, or increased respiratory rate, due to anaemia (p. 17), acidosis (renal failure, p. 5; ketoacidosis of diabetes mellitus, p. 5) and importantly, those cases of dyspnoea or tachypnoea where lung expansion is restricted by the accumulation of pleural fluid. This last group is more important numerically in the cat than the dog. Pericardial effusions may also lead to tachypnoea or dyspnoea, as may pneumonia and some forms of poisoning.

Pleural fluid

Fluid removed from the pleural cavity by thoracentesis (Appendix 1.7) may be classified as blood, chylous fluid, a transudate or an exudate. The appearance of the fluid may be diagnostic.

Blood

Blood, i.e. a sanguineous fluid of similar PCV and haemoglobin concentration to circulating blood, may be due to trauma to the chest, a bleeding neoplasm (haemangiosarcoma) or some defect in haemostasis (*see* p. 19). Pleural blood may well not clot on removal. The loss of blood from the circulation will be reflected in circulatory PCV or haemoglobin concentration only if the loss is chronic, i.e. over 12 hours, and then developing anaemia is usually regenerative in type (p. 17).

Chylous fluid

Chylothorax is seen following trauma or erosion of the thoracic duct; the fluid is milky, heavy in fat and contains large numbers of lymphocytes. A chylous effusion is sometimes seen with anterior mediastinal (thymic) lymphosarcoma in the cat.

Transudates

True thoracic transudates (watery fluids, acellular and with less than 30 g/l protein) are uncommon; where present, their aetiology is similar to true peritoneal transudates (*see* Ascites, p. 9). Modified transudates, which are frequently opaque and blood-tinged, are more common and result from congestive heart failure (particularly in the cat), incarcerated liver from rupture of the diaphragm, or thoracic neoplasia. Pulmonary carcinoma in the cat, though uncommon, characteristically causes such a pleural effusion.

Further examination of the fluid may not distinguish its cause, with the important exceptions of anterior mediastinal lymphosarcoma in the cat, where a smear reveals many lymphocytes (of which some may be lymphoblasts), and the rare cases of mesothelioma, where the experienced cytologist may distinguish neoplastic cells.

Exudates

Thoracic exudates are frequently, though not always, purulent in appearance, and are often referred to as pyothorax. Examination of a smear reveals cellular material (mainly neutrophils) and bacteria. Nocardial effusions often contain cream-coloured granules, which when crushed and stained are rich in organisms. Bacterial culture is valuable to identify the pathogen and, more importantly, its antibiotic sensitivity. Culture, however, may prove negative. The inflammatory response in the pleura will be reflected in a neutrophilia on haematological examination. Some 20 per cent of the cases of feline infectious peritonitis (FIP) will have some pleural effusion and, rarely, some cases may show only pleural fluid. The nature of the fluid and the other laboratory findings in FIP are discussed under Ascites (p. 9).

Pericardial fluid

Congestive heart failure, and the resultant dyspnoea, can follow the accumulation of pericardial fluid. Though the fluid may form as an extension of pleural disease (as in the case of FIP, as part of a polyserositis) it is, in the dog, frequently sanguineous when sampled by pericardiocentesis (Appendix 1.8). Unlike cardiovascular blood, however, it does not clot on standing. Further examination of the fluid is not helpful in differentiating between a pericardial neoplasm, e.g. haemangiosarcoma, or an idiopathic pericardial effusion.

Pneumonia

Where dyspnoea is due to a pneumonia, the only laboratory finding of note is a neutrophilia, except in the rare cases of eosinophilic pneumonia where circulating eosinophil numbers are increased (greater than $1000/\mu l$).

Poisoning

Paraquat, which causes a progressive and inevitably fatal tachypnoea and dyspnoea, may be detected in the urine of dogs for a few days following ingestion but is usually absent by the time the signs are marked. There is no other readily available laboratory test for paraquat.

COUGHING

In neither of the two most common causes of chronic coughing in the dog, i.e. chronic bronchitis or congestive heart failure, is laboratory information of great diagnostic importance. Bacterial culture of tracheal swabs or washings may indicate the antibiotic of choice for treatment of chronic bronchitis. A diagnosis of *Filaroides osleri* infection in young dogs can sometimes be made by the demonstration of larvae in the 'sputum' or faeces, but the results are unreliable and diagnosis is best made or confirmed by bronchoscopy. In the cat *Aleurostrongylus abstrusus* may cause coughing (though the infection is often subclinical) and diagnosis similarly may be made on the demonstration of faeces of the first-stage larvae. In the majority of cases of bronchial asthma in the cat, haematology reveals a marked eosinophilia (15–20 per cent).

ANAEMIA

It is important to remember that anaemia is a clinical sign and not a diagnosis, and definition of the type of anaemia is important if treatment is to be logical. The degree of anaemia, as assessed by the PCV or, perhaps more accurately, by the RBC count or haemoglobin concentration, may not be reflected in the severity of the clinical signs. This is particularly true in the cat, and is related amongst other things to the rate of development of the anaemia. A full haematological profile should be available and anaemia may be divided on this haematological basis (as opposed to aetiological) into regenerative and non-regenerative types.

Regenerative anaemia

Regenerative anaemias are characterized by the appearance of young (larger) red cells and immature red cells (reticulocytes and nucleated red blood cells or normoblasts). The presence of larger red cells amongst the normal mature cells (anisocytosis) is reflected in an increase in the mean corpuscular volume (MCV). The remnants of RNA seen in some young cells stain blue and this is referred to as polychromasia.

Regenerative anaemia may follow blood loss. If blood loss is acute, the real anaemia, i.e. reduction in red cells, is masked haematologically by the hypovolaemia. Blood volume is replaced within 12–24 hours and release of red cells from the marrow reaches a maximum after 3–4 days. Blood lost within the body, e.g. into a serous cavity, is effectively recycled but extracorporeal loss, if longstanding, may lead to iron depletion, seen as microcytosis and a low mean corpuscular haemoglobin concentration (MCHC). Where no evidence of blood loss can be found, further laboratory tests that may help in establishing the cause of the regenerative anaemia include the demonstration of red cell parasites, testing for the presence of feline leukaemia virus (FeLV) infection in the cat and tests for autoimmune disease. Testing for red cell parasites, specifically *Haemobartonella felis* in the cat, is based on careful staining of a blood smear with Giemsa; care must be taken not to produce stain artefacts or to mistake Howell–Jolly bodies (nuclear remnants), which are present in small numbers in normal cats, for the protozoal parasites. *Haemobartonella canis* and *Babesia canis* have not been convincingly recorded in the United Kingdom. Demonstration of *H. felis,* i.e. a diagnosis of feline infectious anaemia (FIA), should be followed by examination for FeLV as there is an epidemiological association between the two agents. FeLV may well, however, cause a haemolytic, and hence regenerative, anaemia in its own right. Autoimmune haemolytic anaemias are classically positive to Coombs and Papain tests and, if part of systemic lupus erythematosus (SLE), are associated with the presence of antinuclear antibodies (ANA) in the serum. In SLE, platelets may also be affected leading to a thrombocytopenia; an immune-mediated glomerulonephritis may also be present leading to proteinuria and hypoalbuminaemia. The LE cell test, based on the demonstration of phagocytosis of nuclear material by neutrophils, has been superseded by serological tests such as the ANA tests; these tests, together with the Coombs and Papain tests, are carried out by specialist laboratories. Red cell destruction may also be caused by toxic substances, e.g. methylene blue in cats, acute lead poisoning. In such cases remaining RBCs may show Heinz bodies (denatured haemoglobin) and in the case of lead poisoning, basophilic stippling of RBC may be present.

If the haemolytic process is rapid enough, for whatever cause, the animal may show haemoglobinuria and/or jaundice. Haemoglobin in urine will react with routine tests for haematuria, being distinguished by examination of urine sediment for RBC. Haemolytic jaundice, being prehepatic, is characterized by unconjugated (indirect reacting) bilirubin. A profound haemolytic jaundice may be seen following an incompatible blood transfusion.

Non-regenerative anaemia

Non-regenerative anaemias (hypoplastic or aplastic) are characterized haematologically by reduced numbers of normal RBC and no evidence of marrow response. The depression of bone-marrow activity may follow intercurrent disease (e.g. chronic renal failure), toxic substances (e.g. oestrogen, chloramphenicol), viral infection (e.g. FeLV) or longstanding bacterial disease. The number of platelets and WBC may also be reduced. The further laboratory investigation of depression anaemias should include measurement of blood urea or creatinine, in the cat testing for FeLV, and bone-marrow biopsy (Appendix 1.9). Interpretation of bone-marrow smears, however, requires some experience.

Nutritional anaemias, where the marrow lacks some raw material for

RBC production, are uncommon. Iron deficiency following chronic blood loss, and folic acid or vitamin B_6 deficiency associated with mal-absorption have been recorded.

HAEMORRHAGE

The investigation of unexplained haemorrhage, either persistent from one site or as multiple ecchymotic lesions, is initially based on distinguishing platelet from clotting factor dysfunction.

Platelet disorders

A crude assessment of platelet numbers and or function may be based on the bleeding time, measured following a small incision in the surface of the ear pinna (Appendix 1.10). Normal bleeding time varies considerably but a time of greater than 5 min can be considered prolonged. Poor clot retraction in a clotted blood sample left to stand on the bench is also an indication of reduced platelet function (a normal clot retracts in 1 hour at 37 °C). More specifically, platelet numbers may be assessed in a blood smear or counted in a haemocytometer. Reduction in platelet numbers may be associated with their destruction in the circulation by immune mechanisms, e.g. idiopathic thrombocytopenia (ITP), systemic lupus erythematosus (SLE). In the latter example, an immune-mediated anaemia (regenerative in type) may also be present and Coombs and anti-nuclear antibody tests will be positive. Reduced production of platelets following bone-marrow suppression may be associated with reductions in RBC and WBC numbers, as in bone-marrow replacement by haemopoietic neo-plasia. A bone-marrow biopsy is useful in such cases.

Disorders of clotting factors

Haemorrhage due to deficiencies in clotting factors, rather than platelet function, is characterized by a prolonged whole blood clotting time. This is measured on a cleanly taken blood sample held at 37 °C (ideally in a water bath, but more crudely in the palm of one's hand) in a glass con-tainer. A time of greater than 12 min is considered abnormal; in platelet dysfunction, clotting time is often reduced (normal 6–12 min). In practice, the demonstration of a prolonged whole blood clotting time together with an appropriate history justifies a presumptive diagnosis of Warfarin poisoning and the use of vitamin K. The more precise definition of clot-ting factor disorders has been well described and may be carried out by specialist laboratories to diagnose the rare cases of haemophilia, von Willebrand's disease and disseminated intravascular coagulation (DIC). It is also worth restating that a number of clotting factors are produced in the liver and that hepatic failure may lead to a prolonged whole blood clotting time and may on occasions be associated with ecchymotic haemorrhages. The laboratory assessment of liver function is discussed elsewhere (p. 11).

EXERCISE INTOLERANCE AND COLLAPSE

The clinical signs of exercise intolerance and collapse are frequently encountered in small animal practice and the cause is often relatively clear, or becomes so using diagnostic aids such as radiography or electro-cardiography (e.g. chronic arthritis, cardiac insufficiency of one cause or another, acute blood loss). There are, however, a number of conditions, some of them obscure, where laboratory data may be helpful, and hence a number of tests that may be applied when the diagnosis is less apparent.

Blood glucose

Blood glucose is low (less than 2·5 mmol/l) in cases of insulinoma: the tumour is seen in older, usually brachycephalic, dogs and cases typically present with incoordination and collapse on exertion and, occasionally, fits. Additional information may be obtained from a glucose tolerance test (Appendix 1.11), where blood glucose levels remain low or rise only transiently following oral glucose, but confirmation of the diagnosis requires a laparotomy. Low blood glucose levels at exercise also lead to collapse in the rare glycogen-storage diseases recorded in working dogs.

Blood electrolytes

High blood potassium (greater than 5·5 mmol/l), together with lower than normal blood sodium (less than 135 mmol/l), often expressed as a Na : K ratio of less than 27:1, is seen in hypoadrenocorticalism (Addison's disease) where reduction in blood pressure may lead to collapse, particularly associated with stress. Blood urea and creatinine levels may be elevated (a pre-renal failure). Blood glucose is sometimes reduced and haematology may reveal eosinophilia and lymphocytosis. Confirmation rests on the lack of response in plasma cortisol levels to stimulation of the adrenals with ACTH.

Creatine phosphokinase

The finding of elevated levels of plasma creatine phosphokinase (CPK) indicates skeletal (or cardiac) muscle degeneration and may be associated with various myopathies and hence, with an inability to exercise. A specific diagnosis rests on muscle biopsy. The degree of elevation of CPK is often dramatic (up to 50 times the normal value of <40 i.u./l) but marked elevations may also occur following exercise and muscle trauma.

In view of this, mild elevations must be interpreted with caution. The division of total CPK values into isoenzymes is potentially useful but is not at present readily available. CPK activity is rapidly lost on storage of samples and so estimations are best made within 24 hours.

There is no elevation in CPK, nor is there any other useful biochemical test, in cases of myasthenia gravis. Diagnosis in such cases is based on the response to an anticholinesterase, either the short-acting edrophonium chloride* or neostigmine.

Haemoglobin

Abnormalities of haemoglobin affecting the efficiency of oxygen carriage have been recorded in the dog as a cause of exercise intolerance or collapse. Such cases are rarely recognized and require detailed laboratory examination for confirmation of the diagnosis. Haemoglobin levels are normal or may be elevated on routine examination.

A distinction may be made between exercise intolerance, or an inability to exercise, and an unwillingness to exercise, or lethargy. The distinction is not always useful; for example, the owner of an Addisonian dog may primarily complain of its lethargy, and lethargy may indeed be associated with any disease state, but a few conditions can be said to show marked lethargy and their diagnosis or exclusion from the differential list may be aided by laboratory tests.

A high blood cholesterol level (greater than 8·0 mmol/l) is a useful, though not specific, indicator of hypothyroidism (cholesterol is also raised in glomerulonephritis, diabetes mellitus and some forms of liver disease). Measurement of circulating thyroid hormone levels or plasma bound iodine (PBI), while possible, is expensive and the results are difficult to interpret: a diagnosis of hypothyroidism is best confirmed by biopsy or on a marked response to hormone replacement therapy. Lethargy is also a feature of hyperadrenocorticalism (Cushing's syndrome), the laboratory investigation of which is covered elsewhere (p. 8). Cases of congenital vascular anomalies of the liver (portasystemic shunts) may show a profound lethargy associated with high levels of blood ammonia (*see also* p. 7 and 11).

HAEMATURIA

Haematuria is frequently a visual rather than a laboratory diagnosis. Haemastix† and the examination of urine sediment will confirm the clinical impression and the latter will distinguish it from the less common haemoglobinuria. Further examination of urine sediment for inflammatory

---

*Tensilon, Roche Products Ltd, Welwyn Garden City, Herts.
†Haemastix, Ames Co., Division of Miles Laboratories Ltd, Slough, Berks.

cells (WBC) and bacteria will help to establish the presence of urinary tract infection, of which bladder infection, cystitis, is the commonest cause of haematuria. Such results should be followed by urine culture and sensitivity testing. Less commonly, prostatic bleeding may lead to haematuria, or blood may be renal in origin, e.g. following renal trauma, or in rare cases of renal carcinoma. Renal carcinoma may be also associated with polycythaemia (increase in RBC numbers) due to excessive production of erythropoietin.

ATAXIA

Many of the causes of ataxia may be classed as surgical (e.g. cervical spine instability), congenital abnormalities (e.g. feline ataxia, lysosomal storage disease) or toxic (e.g. alpha-chloralose or metaldehyde poisoning), and as such are largely unsuited to laboratory investigation, at least of a routine nature.

Ataxia may also result from hypoglycaemia, due usually to hyper-insulinism — either iatrogenic or from an insulinoma (*see also* p. 20) — or to hypocalcaemia, e.g. lactation tetany or eclampsia. Both conditions progress to muscle twitching, fits and eventual coma.

POOR GROWTH OR WEIGHT LOSS

In the absence of an obvious cause for poor growth in the young dog or cat, e.g. malnutrition, heavy parasitic infestation, persistent regurgitation or diarrhoea, laboratory investigation should include an assessment of renal and hepatic function. Cases of congenital renal disease show the biochemical and haematological changes of chronic renal failure (p. 5) while cases of congenital vascular anomalies of the liver (porta-caval or portasystemic shunts) present as chronic hepatic failure (p. 11). Where the anomalous portal vessel(s) is large, e.g. patent ductus venosus, portal hypertension may not occur and thus no ascites forms; the increase in blood ammonia levels, however (and thus clinical signs of hepatic encephalopathy), may be marked in such cases.

Animals presenting with weight loss as the major clinical signs should also be assessed for renal and hepatic function. Laboratory tests are generally of less help in neoplastic disease, clinical examination or other diagnostic aids such as radiography being more useful. Exceptions include the demonstration of obstructive jaundice in pancreatic carcinoma (*see* p. 13), reduced xylose absorption in alimentary lymphosarcoma (*see* p. 3), the presence of feline leukaemia virus (FeLV) in the cat and the use of haematology and bone-marrow biopsy in haemopoietic neoplasia. A neutrophilia may be present in neoplastic disease associated with tumour necrosis. Haemopoietic neoplasms may be divided into myeloid, which are uncommon but more frequently truly leukaemic, and lymphoid neoplasms, the latter typically presenting with tumour formation. Anaemia, either regenerative or non-regenerative, is the most consistent haematological finding in haemopoietic neoplasia but in the absence of abnormal circulating blood cells or discrete tumours a definitive diagnosis relies on the examination of bone-marrow smears (Appendix 1.9).

PYREXIA

Pyrexia is a frequent clinical sign most commonly associated with acute viral or bacterial infections and as such is usually accompanied by other clinical signs. Where pyrexia persists and is unexplained, i.e. a pyrexia of unknown origin (PUO), certain laboratory tests may be helpful. Haematological examination may reveal a neutrophilia, though the inflammatory response this represents may be immune-mediated (e.g. systemic lupus erythematosus), infectious (e.g. bacterial endocarditis) and non-infectious (e.g. feline pansteatitis tumour necrosis) in origin. The laboratory investigation of autoimmune disease has been covered elsewhere (*see* p. 18). The diagnosis of bacterial endocarditis relies on the isolation of the causative organism from the blood. This should be attempted, using special culture media, during periods of pyrexia and before antibiotic treatment has been started. Positive cultures are, however, difficult to obtain even when serial samples are taken. The presence of pansteatitis is confirmed by biopsy of subcutaneous fat. Recurrent pyrexia is occasionally seen associated with portovascular anomalies in young dogs (*see* p. 11).

REFERENCE

Bush B. M. (1975) *Veterinary Laboratory Manual.* London, Heinemann Medical.

Chapter 2

Surgical Pathology

I: The Skin
II: The Mammary Glands

The purpose of Chapters 2 and 3 is to provide the small animal clinician with an outline of the common and important neoplasms arising in the skin (Part I) and in its associated structures, including the mammary gland (Part II). Emphasis is placed on the clinicopathological aspects of these tumours — their prevalence, site of occurrence, breed and age incidence and their behaviour and treatment. Texts that provide inclusive cover of all types of skin and mammary neoplasms are available (Bostock and Owen, 1975; Moulton, 1978), but most have been written with the pathologist in mind so that their emphasis is on the microscopic appearances of tumours rather than on their clinical behaviour.

It cannot be stressed too strongly that close co-operation between the clinician and pathologist is essential if anything of real value is to be obtained from the examination of biopsy material. This requires complete and accurate documentation of the material by the clinician and a useful report from the pathologist on which the clinician can base his management of the case.

The clinician should provide the following information:

Breed, age and sex of the animal.

Site, size and duration of lesion(s).

Presence or absence of local lymph node enlargement.

Details of any treatment.

Previous occurrence of the tumour.

Last oestrus period in case of mammary tumours.

Owner references (name, address).

Specimens should be submitted whole, where possible, in a *wide-necked* container full of formalin (*see* Appendix 2 for details). The container lid should be secure to prevent leaking, and the specimen wrapped and posted to comply with current Post Office regulations (*see* Appendix

3). If the entire specimen is too large then a good representative sample should be sent. This should include viable tumour and the junction between it and the adjacent normal tissues. It is always important to include some surrounding normal tissue since the pathologist can then give information about the adequacy of removal.

The *pathologist* should report the following information:

A detailed gross and histological description of the lesion.

A diagnosis.

An assessment of whether excision is complete.

An indication of the likely behaviour of the tumour where this is not well known.

Both clinician and pathologist should cooperate in providing as complete a follow-up history as possible. This is essential if we are to increase our understanding of tumour behaviour. Furthermore, information of this sort is the only way in which pathologists can learn about their diagnostic errors and so increase their competence.

INCIDENCE OF TUMOURS

Until recently it was not possible to say what the true incidence of a particular animal tumour was, since no carefully analysed population-based studies of cancer in animals had been made. Collections of neoplasms reported from veterinary schools took no account of the population from which they were drawn. Furthermore, they tended to be a biased selection through referral and because of the specific interests of the members of the departments concerned in their collection. During the past decade, however, schemes have developed with the aim of collecting and collating data on tumours from a number of veterinary pathology centres. One of the largest schemes is the Veterinary Medical Data Program (VMDP) which utilizes data collected from twelve colleges of veterinary medicine in the United States of America and Canada (Priester, 1973). A similar scheme operates in Alameda County, California where a population-based animal tumour registry has operated since 1963 (Dorn et al., 1968; Schneider, 1975). Such schemes have not only provided valuable and reliable information about the prevalence of tumours in animals but also have indicated the distribution and frequency of tumour types among the species and the risk factors related to their development.

The information given in these two chapters is based partly on the author's own experience and partly on published reports. Some of the observations may be contentious since they have not been derived from the sort of statistical analysis that occurs in the VMDP. The cat and the dog will be dealt with separately and, although this means that a number of neoplasms will be mentioned twice, it nevertheless serves to emphasize their differing importance and behaviour in each of the species.

I: The Skin

SKIN TUMOURS IN THE CAT

Incidence

Figures taken from the VMDP (Priester, 1973) and the Alameda County
tumour registry (Dorn et al., 1968) put the incidence of skin neoplasia in
the cat at 18 per cent and 44 per cent of all tumours, respectively. This is a
surprisingly wide discrepancy and it is interesting that the incidence of
feline skin neoplasia in a series reported from the University of
Pennsylvania closely parallels that of the VMDP. It would appear, therefore,
that skin tumours in the cat probably account for about 20 per cent of all
tumours that occur in this species. Of these skin tumours, 40 per cent are
malignant.

Age, sex and breed incidence

With the exception of the fibrosarcoma, which may occur in young
cats, the other skin neoplasms appear in the adult or aged animal.
Ceruminous gland tumours of the ear canal have been reported to occur
predominantly in aged cats (Cotchin, 1961) while the other tumours
discussed below usually appear at any age from 5 years upwards.

There does not appear to be any particular breed or sex incidence of
skin tumours in the cat.

Types of tumour

There is not nearly such a wide variety of histological types of skin tumour
in the cat as in the dog. Those that will be considered are:
Epithelial neoplasms
Adnexal tumours (including ceruminous gland tumours of the ear).
Squamous cell carcinoma.
Mesenchymal neoplasms
Fibrous tissue tumours.
Mast cell tumours.
Under the heading of adnexal tumours are included tumours that arise
from the basal layer of the epidermis, the hair follicles, the sweat,
sebaceous and ceruminous glands. In the cat adnexal tumours are one of
the most common types of skin tumour. They arise chiefly from two sites,
the basal layer of the epidermis and the ceruminous glands of the ear
canal.

Adnexal tumours (basal cell origin)

Site and gross appearance. Most occur around the face (particularly near
the base of the ear), neck and over the trunk. They are usually solitary,

well demarcated, discrete masses of up to 4 cm diameter. Some are cystic. The overlying epidermis may be thin and hairless or ulcerated. They are frequently heavily pigmented and may be mistaken for melanomas which are very rare tumours in the cat.

Behaviour and treatment. Most are slow growing, do not infiltrate the local tissues and do not metastasize. Surgical removal or cryosurgery are the best methods of treatment and in most cases carry an excellent prognosis.

Adnexal tumours (ceruminous gland)

Site and gross appearance. These tumours arise in the horizontal ear canal, particularly in its deeper parts. The smaller, nodular masses must be differentiated from otitis externa for which they may be mistaken. Larger, pedunculated tumours are frequently ulcerated and some may infiltrate the cartilage of the ear canal and form a large ulcerating mass at the base of the ear. Pedunculated tumours must be differentiated from inflammatory polyps which arise in the middle ear.

Behaviour and treatment. Almost 50 per cent of ceruminous gland tumours are malignant. They tend to recur after removal and will invade the parotid region and metastasize to the parotid lymph node. Excision seems to be the only treatment of any value.

Squamous cell carcinoma

Site and gross appearance. This is one of the most common skin tumours of the cat. It occurs almost invariably in the head region, especially in areas of unpigmented skin, so that the white cat is particularly at risk. Sites of predilection are the tips of the pinnae (*Fig.* 2.1), the nasal planum, external nares (*Fig.* 2.2), eyelids and lips.

The tumours on the ears often develop insidiously over many months, first appearing as scaling areas of hair loss on the tips and margins of the pinna, later progressing to a crusted ulcerated lesion which eventually may invade the auricular cartilage and cause severe destruction of the ear. In the early stages they are often mistaken for eczematous, parasitic or traumatic lesions.

At other sites the squamous cell carcinoma appears as a small erosive, non-healing, ulcerated lesion with a firm raised edge. It may be confused with eosinophilic granuloma when it occurs on the lips or nose.

Behaviour and treatment. Most of these tumours can be cured by radical excision but if excision is incomplete they will recur. They are locally invasive but slow to metastasize to the regional lymph nodes. Cryosurgery is particularly useful when tumours occur on the eyelids, nasal planum or external nares.

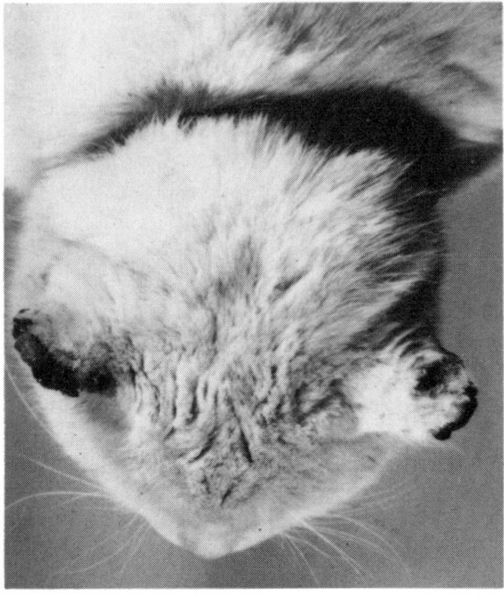

Fig. 2.1. Squamous cell carcinoma on the tips of the ears of a white cat.

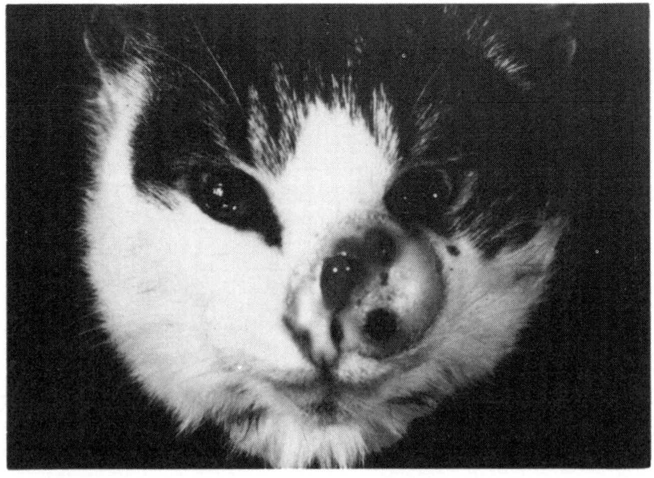

Fig. 2.2. Squamous cell carcinoma of the external nares. The adjacent epithelial
surface is stretched and ulcerated by the underlying invasive carcinoma.

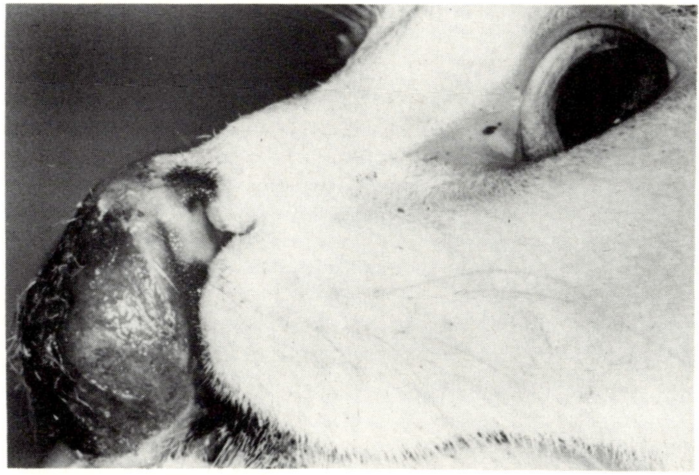

Fig. 2.3. Fibrosarcoma on the external nares of a 2-year-old cat.

Fibrous tissue tumours

Site and gross appearance. These tumours arise in the subcutis and occur particularly on the limbs and head. They are firm, ill-defined, nodular tumours which are frequently ulcerated. Cut surfaces reveal firm yellow–white tissue, often with a characteristic whorled pattern.

Behaviour and treatment. Although benign tumours of fibrous tissue (fibromas) are described in the cat, the author's experience suggests that these are exceedingly rare and that most tumours should be regarded as fibrosarcomas. They are locally invasive and may be difficult to delineate so that wide excision is necessary. They may occur in young animals (*Fig.* 2.3). There is a marked tendency for these tumours to recur and some ultimately metastasize. X-irradiation appears to be of little value in their treatment. Amputation of affected limbs is the treatment of choice where radical excision may be difficult.

Mast cell tumours

These are the least common of the feline skin tumours discussed here and, although they are said to account for approximately 2–3 per cent of all cutaneous tumours in the cat (Moulton, 1978), they are, in the author's experience, very unusual.

Site and gross appearance. The tumours tend to be small (up to 0·5 cm in diameter), multiple and to involve the head and neck particularly. They are usually discrete, firm yellow–white nodules in the subcutis; there may be ulceration of overlying skin.

Behaviour and treatment. Prognosis for feline mast cell tumours should be guarded because of the frequency with which they spread to regional lymph nodes and internal organs.

NON-NEOPLASTIC TUMOUR-LIKE LESIONS OF THE SKIN
IN THE CAT

There are always a number of lesions removed from the skin which the clinician believes to be neoplastic but which on subsequent histological examination prove otherwise. Most of these lesions are found to be of an inflammatory nature. The most common in the cat are:

Eosinophilic granuloma complex.

Feline leprosy.

Eosinophilic granuloma complex

This complex consists of three distinct chronic inflammatory lesions of unknown cause:

Eosinophilic ulcer (rodent ulcer). This lesion is seen most commonly on the upper lip (*Fig.* 2.4) but also at the angle of the jaw and occasionally in the mouth, on the tongue and on the neck and thighs. It is a raised, red–brown ulcerated lesion that may be mistaken for a squamous cell carcinoma when it occurs on the lips (although it is generally found in a younger age group of cats).

Eosinophilic plaque (granuloma, feline lick granuloma). Lesions occur most frequently on the abdomen and back. They are raised, discrete, plaque-like ulcers and are associated with excessive licking and chewing. They occur in younger cats than do eosinophilic ulcers.

Linear eosinophilic granuloma. Most cats affected are less than 1 year old so that confusion with neoplasia seems unlikely. The lesions occur mainly on the posterior aspect of the hind legs or on the medial surface of the forelegs. They are raised, firm, cord-like dermal masses that appear slightly pink but they are usually not ulcerated.

Treatment. All three types of lesion are said to respond to systemic corticosteroid therapy although surgery or cryosurgery may be required in certain cases.

Feline leprosy

This condition is not seen as frequently as the eosinophilic granuloma complex. Cats of any age, breed or sex may be affected. The lesions occur as firm, discrete, spherical nodules (up to 2 cm in diameter) in the subcutaneous tissues, particularly around the head and limbs. They tend to enlarge slowly and frequently the surface is ulcerated.

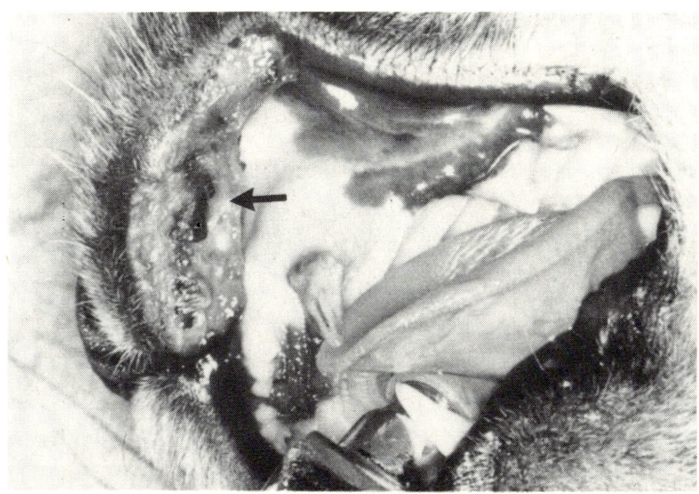

Fig. 2.4. Eosinophilic ulcer (arrow) on the lip margin of a cat.

Histologically the lesions are composed of granulomatous collections of macrophages filled with numerous acid- and alcohol-fast bacilli. In spite of this it is often not possible to culture and identify the organisms although in some cases *Mycobacterium lepraemurium,* the rat leprosy bacillus, has been isolated and in others *Mycobacterium fortuitum* has been cultured (Wilkinson et al., 1978). The presence of these organisms in impression smears from the lesions can be used as a diagnostic aid.

Treatment. Surgical excision is the only course. There is no indication that the condition can spread to man, a feature that obviously concerns an owner when told of the diagnosis.

SKIN TUMOURS IN THE DOG

Incidence

The skin is by far the commonest site for neoplasia in the dog, accounting for 28 per cent (Priester, 1973) to 35·6 per cent (Brodey, 1970) of all tumours in this species. Approximately 20 per cent of canine skin tumours are malignant, half the figure for skin malignancy in the cat (Priester and Mantel, 1971).

Age

With the exception of the histiocytoma, 75 per cent of which occur in animals less than 3 years old, most skin tumours in the dog appear in older animals.

Breed

Unlike the cat, the dog shows a distinct breed incidence of certain types of skin tumour. These are listed in Tables 2.1 and 2.2 and are also indicated in the description of each type of tumour.

Sex

There is some indication that mesenchymal tumours (e.g. lipomas and mast cell tumours) are more common in bitches than in dogs (Priester and Mantel, 1971). It is also well known that perianal gland tumours occur almost exclusively in males.

Types

The dog has the widest range of histological types of skin tumour of all the domestic species. About 45 per cent are of epithelial origin, 50 per cent of mesenchymal origin and the remaining 5 per cent are melanotic tumours.

    Epithelial neoplasms
        Adnexal tumours.
        Perianal gland tumours.
        Squamous cell carcinomas.
    Mesenchymal neoplasms
        Mast cell tumours.
        Lipomas.
        Haemangiopericytoma.
        Histiocytoma.
        Vascular tumours.
        Fibrous tissue tumours.
    Melanotic neoplasms

Adnexal tumours

These tumours, which are derived from a variety of the skin adnexae, are grouped under one heading since they are often of mixed cellular type and most are benign. They are very common in the dog.

    Sites and gross appearance. Tumours of sebaceous gland, hair follicle and basal cell origin are found predominantly in the head (often on the eyelids) (*Fig.* 2.5) and neck region while those derived from sweat glands occur chiefly on the trunk. They are well-circumscribed, bulging tumours that may become ulcerated. The sebaceous gland tumours have waxy, friable cut surfaces; those of hair follicle origin frequently contain small cysts filled with white keratin and the sweat gland tumours are often cystic.

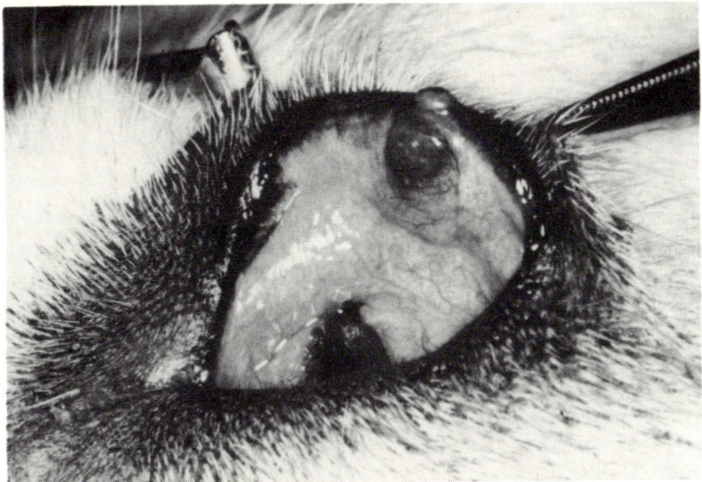

Fig. 2.5. Pigmented adnexal tumour on the palpebral margin of a 9-year-old Labrador dog.

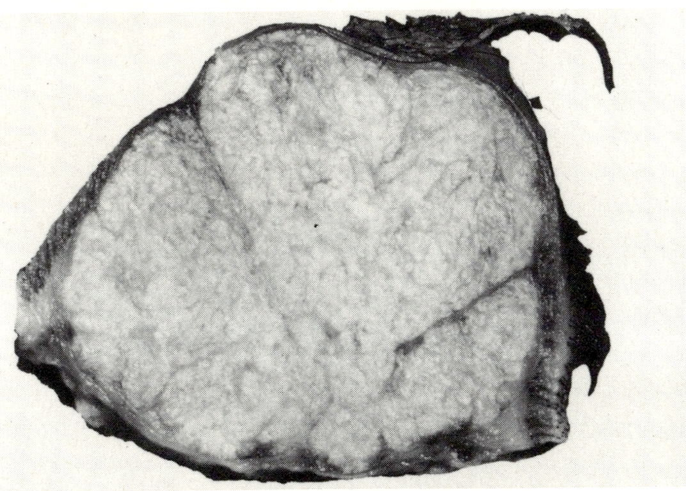

Fig. 2.6. Calcifying epithelioma in a Kerry Blue dog.

Breed incidence. The Cocker Spaniel is predisposed to adnexal tumours of sebaceous and basal cell origin. The Kerry Blue (and probably the Poodle) are particularly prone to tumours of hair follicle origin (*Fig.* 2.6).

Behaviour and treatment. Since the great majority of these tumours are benign, surgical removal is curative. Cryosurgery is particularly useful at sites such as the eyelid where scar tissue is disfiguring.

Table 2.1. Skin tumours of the dog: benign clinical features

Descriptive term	Age	Site(s)	Gross appearance	Suggested breed & sex prevalence	Behaviour & treatment
Adnexal† tumours:*					
Sebaceous tumour	Old	Head & neck	Bulging, well-circumscribed waxy, friable surfaces	Cocker Spaniel	Grow slowly. Most show expansile rather than in-filtrative growth. No recurrence if completely excised
Basal cell tumour	Mature	Head & neck	Bulging, well-circumscribed may be ulcerated	Cocker Spaniel	
Hair follicle tumour	Mature	Head & neck	Bulging cysts filled with white keratin	Kerry Blue, Poodle	
Sweat gland tumour	Mature	Trunk	Bulging, often cystic		
Perianal* gland tumour	Mature/ old	Perianal, tail, prepuce and back	Bulging, rubbery, ulcerated. Poorly delineated. May be multiple	Spaniel (almost always in males)	May grow very large. Temporary regression with Stilboestrol therapy or castration, but may be useful adjunct to surgery. Surgery treatment of choice.
Melanoma*	Old	Hairy skin at any site	Pedunculated, polypoid or dome-shaped. Rubbery and heavily pigmented	Darker Breeds (e.g. Airedale, Scottie, Cocker Spaniel)	Slow growing. No recurrence if completely excised
Lipoma*	Old	Chest, axilla, flank & groin	Well-circumscribed, soft, yellow–white and greasy	Obese bitches	Grow very slowly, may be multiple
Histio-cytoma*	Young (75%< 3 yr)	Head (especially pinna)	Dome-shaped, ulcerated well-defined, pale, firm cut surfaces	Boxer, Dachshund	Grow rapidly. Regress spontaneously in 3–6 months but usually excised
Haeman-gioma	Old		Fluctuating, bulging Haemorrhagic cut surfaces	Boxer	Fluctuating growth because of haemorrhage. Surgical excision is curative
Fibroma	Old		Dome-shaped, firm whorled pale surfaces		Slow growing. No recurrence if completely excised

* Commonly occurring benign tumours
† Many adnexal tumours are of mixed histological type

Table 2.2. Skin tumours of the dog: malignant clinical features

Descriptive term	Age	Site(s)	Gross appearance	Suggested breed & sex prevalence	Behaviour & treatment
Squamous cell carcinoma	Old	Limbs, digits and trunk	Indurated, ulcerated, will invade bone of digits		Slow-growing, locally invasive. Slow to metastasize. Radical excision or amputation of digits gives a good prognosis
Melanoma	Old	Scrotum, digits and lips	Ulcerated, ill-defined variable pigmentation	Darker breeds	Tend to grow rapidly. Locally invasive with local and distant metastasis. Prognosis guarded after excision
Mast cell* tumour	Mature	Thigh, trunk & scrotum	Slow-growing: well-defined, soft yellowish. Rapidly growing: ulcerated, ill-defined yellow & haemorrhagic	Boxer, Labrador, Retriever, Bull Terrier and Boston Terrier	Well-differentiated tumours surgically cured in approximately 80% of animals. Poorly differentiated tumours recur after removal and metastasize
Haemangio-* pericytoma	Old	Forelegs & thighs	Firm, nodular bulging masses, rarely ulcerated	Boxer, Alsatian, Cocker & Springer Spaniel	Slow growing. Often difficult to remove completely. Tend to recur but rarely metastasize
Haemangio-sarcoma	Old		Large ulcerated, haemorrhagic & cystic	Alsatians	Aggressive, rapidly growing. Metastases common. Prognosis poor.
Fibrosar-coma	Young		Bulging, ulcerated. Poorly delineated, lobulated firm yellow–white cut surfaces		Locally invasive. Tend to recur after removal. May metastasize. Amputation may be treatment of choice. X-irradiation may help

*Commonly occurring locally aggressive or malignant tumours

Perianal gland tumours (Hepatoid gland tumours)

These tumours are peculiar to the dog and occur almost exclusively in the male. They are among the most common types of skin tumour in this species.

Sites and gross appearance. Perianal gland tumours occur not only in the perianal region but can arise on the tail, the prepuce, perineum and occasionally on the back. They are bulging, rubbery tumours which are frequently ulcerated and may be difficult to delineate. They may occur at multicentric sites especially in the perianal region.

Breed incidence. The Cocker Spaniel is predisposed to perianal gland tumours.

Behaviour and treatment. Most tumours are benign and do not recur if adequately removed, although they may develop at new sites. They are hormone-dependent tumours and although they will regress temporarily as the result of castration or stilboestrol therapy this treatment alone is not curative. Hormone-induced regression, however, can be useful before surgery in the case of the very large tumours. Perianal gland tumours are radiosensitive and irradiation is said to result in long term regression (Bostock and Owen, 1975). Cryosurgery combined with castration is also a good method of treatment.

Squamous cell carcinoma

Less common than adnexal or perianal gland tumours, the squamous cell carcinoma is, nevertheless, a fairly common skin tumour in the dog.

Sites and gross appearance. Squamous cell carcinomas occur on the limbs, the digits and the trunk. They are indurated, ulcerated lesions which tend to invade bone when they occur on the digits (*Fig.* 2.7).

Behaviour and treatment. These are locally invasive tumours which are slow to metastasize. Radical excision or (in the case of the digital tumours) amputation is the treatment of choice.

Mast cell tumours

These are one of the most common skin tumours in the dog and because of their potentially malignant behaviour they are, without doubt, the most important of the cutaneous neoplasms in this animal.

Sites and gross appearance. The most common sites are thigh, trunk and scrotum but mast cell tumours can arise anywhere. Multiple tumours are not infrequent. Their gross appearance varies with the rapidity of their growth. Fast-growing tumours are poorly delineated (*Fig.* 2.8), firm, multinodular lesions which frequently invade and ulcerate through the

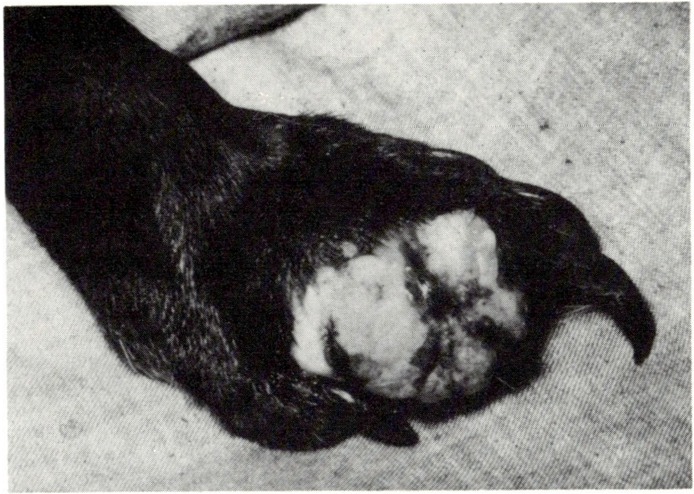

Fig. 2.7. Diffusely spreading and ulcerating squamous cell carcinoma around a nail in a dog.

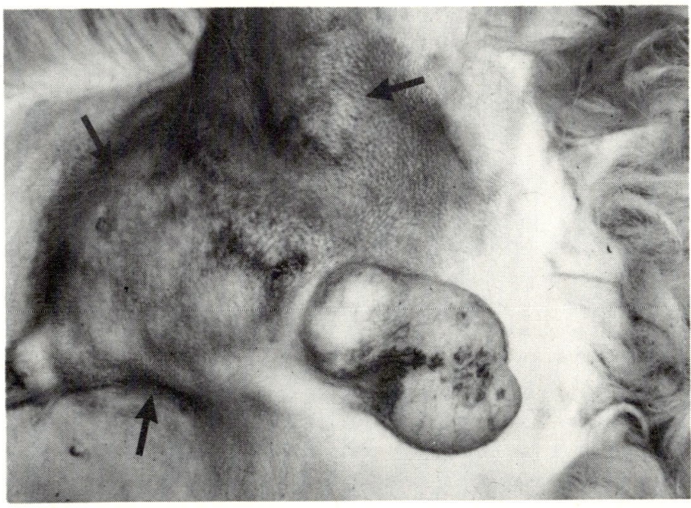

Fig. 2.8. Cutaneous mast cell tumour (arrows) in a dog. There is a diffuse swelling of the skin between the prepuce, scrotum and thigh.

overlying skin. The slower-growing tumours are better defined, rarely ulcerated and usually softer than the more aggressive tumours. The cut surfaces of mast cell tumours are often yellowish, fleshy and oedematous and sometimes mottled by haemorrhage.

Breed incidence. Several breeds of dog are predisposed to the development of mast cell tumours. These include the Boxer, Labrador, Retriever, Bull Terrier, Staffordshire Bull Terrier and the Boston Terrier.

Behaviour and treatment. Bostock (1973) has shown that the degree of differentiation of the neoplastic mast cells is of prognostic value. Poorly differentiated tumours have a marked tendency to recur and to metastasize to local lymph nodes, while slow-growing, well-differentiated tumours are surgically cured in about 80 per cent of animals. In spite of this, it is probably best to regard all mast cell tumours as potentially malignant until the pathologist's report is received. Bostock (1973) has shown that mast cell tumours are radiosensitive and that there can be a significant prolongation of life, even in those dogs with lymph node metastasis. He recommends the use of fractioned X-irradiation to a total tumour dose of 3000–3500 rad.

Other clinical effects of mast cell tumours. Apart from the presence of the tumour itself, in a few cases there are other related clinical problems. The most important of these is the development of peptic ulcers, either in the fundus or pyloric antrum of the stomach or the upper duodenum. The ulcers probably result from gastric hyperacidity caused by histamine release from the mast cell tumours. In many cases the ulcers are too superficial and small to cause any clinical signs but in some cases they become deeply erosive causing pain, anorexia, vomiting, blood loss and anaemia. Occasionally they perforate resulting in fatal haemorrhage or a rapidly developing peritonitis.

Lipomas

These are very common tumours which occur particularly in obese, middle-aged or old bitches.

Sites and gross appearance. Lipomas arise in the subcutaneous tissues of the chest, axilla, flank and groin. They may be solitary or multiple and are soft, mobile tumours which are usually well-circumscribed and finely encapsulated. On section they are composed of soft, yellow–white homogeneous tissue which may contain areas of haemorrhage or chalky white foci of fat necrosis. Lipomas float in formalin fixative.

Behaviour and treatment. Lipomas grow slowly over a long period of time and for this reason many are probably never removed. Lipomas sometimes infiltrate between muscle bundles, especially around the femur, making surgical excision difficult and in these instances recurrence is likely. This type of tumour has been termed 'infiltrative lipoma' (McChesney et al., 1980) and is similar to the tumour of the same name in man. In most cases, however, surgical excision is easy and there is no likelihood of recurrence.

Haemangiopericytoma

This tumour is peculiar to the dog amongst the domestic animals but in spite of its distinctive histological appearance its precise derivation is still not certain.

Sites and gross appearance. These are subcutaneous tumours which occur most commonly on the forelegs (*Fig.* 2.9) and thighs. They are firm, bulging masses with ill-defined edges and can be very large. The skin over the surface is rarely ulcerated. The cut surface is firm, lobulated, grey–pink and may contain mucinous areas.

Breed incidence. Boxers, Alsatians, Cocker and Springer Spaniels all appear to be predisposed to the development of haemangiopericytomas.

Behaviour and treatment. These are slow-growing tumours which may be difficult to remove completely because of their infiltrative nature. Recurrence is common but metastasis is rare. These tumours are not

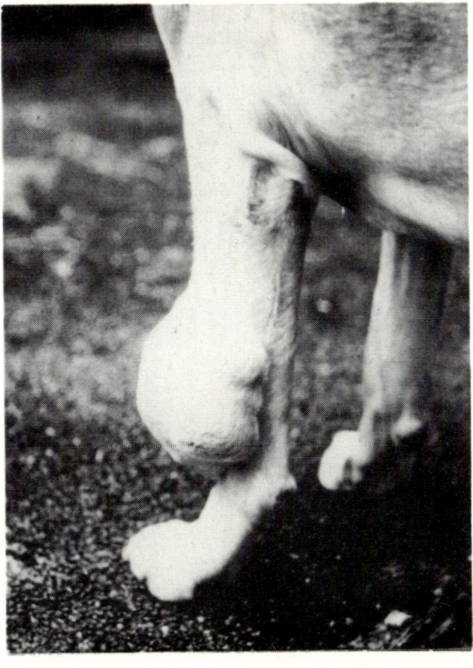

Fig. 2.9. Haemangiopericytoma overlying the radius of a 10-year-old Boxer dog. The intact skin is raised and stretched by the lobulated subcutaneous tumour.

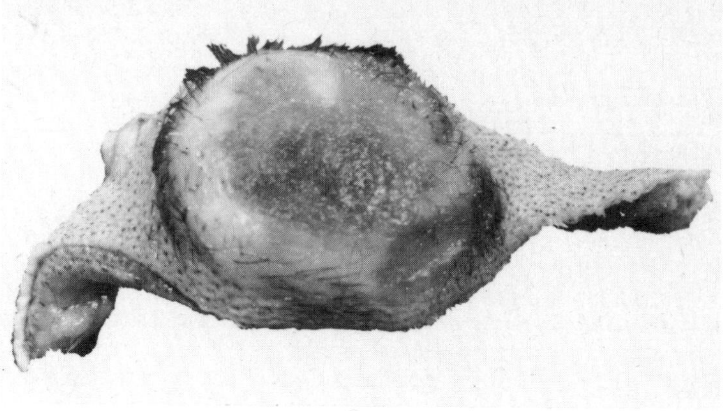

Fig. 2.10. Canine cutaneous histiocytoma. The overlying skin is raised, stretched and ulcerated.

radiosensitive and repeated surgical excision or even amputation may be necessary in some cases.

Histiocytoma

The histiocytoma, like the haemangiopericytoma, is a lesion that occurs only in the dog. It bears no resemblance to the tumour of the same name in man. It is a common cutaneous tumour in the dog and is derived from the monocyte–macrophage series of cells.

Sites and gross appearance. The commonest site is the head, especially on the pinna of the ear. They are usually solitary tumours and seldom grow larger than 2 cm in diameter. They are dome-shaped lesions which are frequently ulcerated but usually free of the underlying tissues (*Fig.* 2.10). On section they appear well-defined but not encapsulated and are composed of firm, homogeneous pale tissue (*Fig.* 2.11).

Age and breed incidence. Histiocytoma is the one skin tumour that characteristically affects young dogs. Approximately 75 per cent occur in dogs less than 3 years old, but they can occur at any age.

There is also some indication of a breed incidence of histiocytomas, with Boxers and Dachshunds appearing to be particularly prone to their development.

Behaviour and treatment. Histiocytomas grow rapidly, often reaching their maximum size within 4 weeks. In spite of this and the high mitotic rate seen microscopically, these are benign tumours which never metastasize. If left, most are said to regress spontaneously within 3–6 months. This regression is associated with infiltration of the tumour by lymphoid

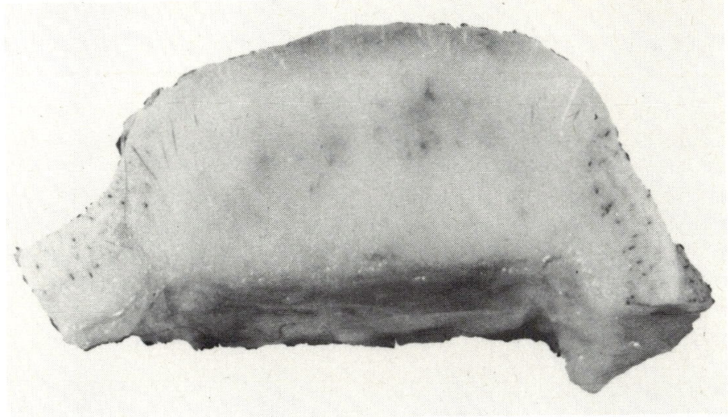

Fig. 2.11. Cut surface of a canine cutaneous histiocytoma, showing the blurring of dermal–epidermal demarcation.

cells which is indicative of an immune-mediated anti-tumour response. So far no aetiological agent has been isolated from histiocytomas although their natural history suggests that they may be of viral origin.

In practice most histiocytomas are removed because of their alarming rate of growth so that the clinician is rarely aware that they may regress spontaneously.

Vascular tumours

Vascular tumours of the skin are less common than the other mesenchymal tumours so far described.

Sites and gross appearance. These lesions can arise at any cutaneous site and they show no particular area of predilection. The tumours form fluctuating bulging masses in the subcutis and have haemorrhagic cut surfaces (*Fig.* 2.12). Benign tumours (haemangiomas) are usually small, while malignant tumours (haemangiosarcomas) are often large and ulcerated.

Breed incidence. Alsatians appear to be predisposed to haemangiosarcomas of the subcutis, while the incidence of haemangiomas in Boxers is higher than expected.

Behaviour and treatment. Haemangiomas do not recur after surgical excision. Haemangiosarcomas are rapidly growing, invasive tumours which recur after removal and tend to metastasize rapidly. They are one of the most aggressive of all the skin tumours in the dog and the prognosis is usually very poor. They are often mistaken for haematomas and treated accordingly.

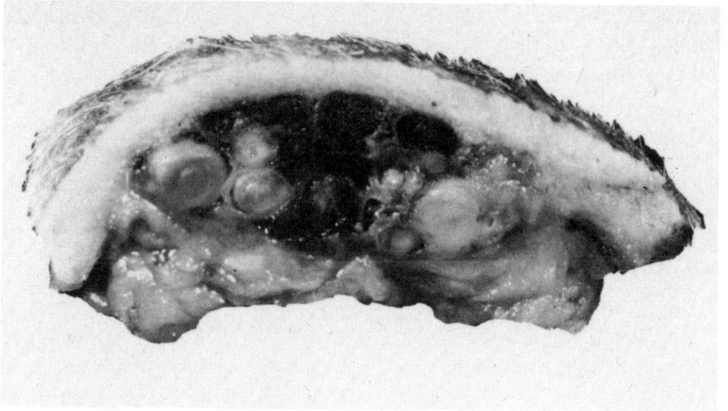

Fig. 2.12. Cut surface of a cavernous dermal haemangioma in a dog.

Fibrous tissue tumours

In the author's experience these are very uncommon cutaneous tumours in
the dog. This observation does not agree with that of some other authors
(Brodey, 1970; Bostock and Owen, 1975) who regard fibrous tissue
tumours of the dermis as quite common in the dog. It seems likely that
this discrepancy, in part, stems from the histological similarity between
fibrous tissue tumours, haemangiopericytomas and, less commonly, neural
tumours, other poorly differentiated sarcomas and nodular fasciitis.

Sites and gross appearance. There does not appear to be any site of
predilection for these tumours. Benign tumours (fibromas) are well-
circumscribed dome-shaped masses which are not usually ulcerated. They
have firm, yellow-white cut surfaces with a distinct whorled pattern.
Fibrosarcomas tend to be larger, ulcerated and poorly delineated. On
section they are lobulated lesions with firm yellow-white areas, softer
pink-grey areas and foci of haemorrhage and necrosis.

Behaviour and treatment. Fibromas are slow growing and do not recur
if completely excised. Fibrosarcomas are rapidly growing invasive tumours
which can occur in very young animals. Surgical removal is often difficult
and they tend to recur and may metastasize. Fibrosarcomas in the dog
appear to be more radiosensitive than in the cat so that surgery followed
by X-irradiation may be curative.

Melanotic neoplasms

These are amongst the more common of the cutaneous neoplasms in the
dog. They are derived from melanin-producing cells which are of neuro-

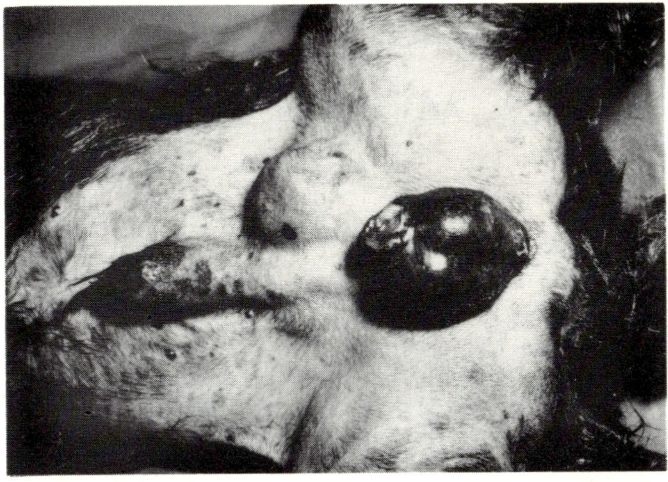

Fig. 2.13. Heavily pigmented scrotal melanoma in a dog. The scrotal surface is ulcerated and a secondary tumour deposit is present beneath the surface of the para-preputial skin.

ectodermal origin and are found between the cells of the basal layer of the epidermis and in the hair bulbs.

Melanomas in the dog behave very differently according to their site of origin (*see below* and Tables 2.1 and 2.2) and it is important that the clinician should be aware of this.

Sites and gross appearance. Benign, slow-growing tumours arise in the hairy skin at any site on the body. They are often pedunculated, polypoid or dome-shaped lesions which are rubbery and heavily pigmented. They may be multiple.

Melanomas arising in the non-hairy skin around the digits, scrotum (*Fig.* 2.13) and lips are often malignant. They tend to grow rapidly, ulcerate and are locally invasive. Pigment may not be obvious on their cut surfaces.

Breed incidence. Melanomas are most frequently seen in dogs with heavily pigmented skin, e.g. Scottie, Airedale and Cocker Spaniel.

Behaviour and treatment. Melanomas of the hairy skin (*see above* and Tables 2.1 and 2.2) are nearly always benign and will not recur after excision. Many are probably never removed because of their slow rate of growth. In contrast, melanomas on the scrotum, lips or around the digits are invasive, malignant tumours which tend to recur after removal and will metastasize. Amputation of affected digits is recommended and at the other sites of malignancy X-irradiation may be a useful adjunct to surgery, but the prognosis should always be guarded.

NON-NEOPLASTIC TUMOUR-LIKE LESIONS OF THE SKIN
IN THE DOG

As in the cat, there are always a number of cutaneous masses which are not neoplastic but which are thought by the clinician at the time of surgery to be tumours.

The most important of these lesions are:

Cysts.

Calcinosis circumscripta.

Lick granuloma.

Cysts

Epidermoid and dermoid cysts arise fairly commonly in the dermis over the trunk of older dogs. They may be multiple and usually do not grow much larger than 3 cm in diameter. They are well-circumscribed lesions which have a thick wall and contain laminated white material or turbid fluid. The cysts are lined by stratified squamous epithelium and contain keratin (epidermoid) and sometimes fragments of hair (dermoid). If the cysts rupture, releasing their contents into the surrounding dermis, then an intense inflammatory reaction results and the lesion may become ulcerated.

Treatment. Cysts will not recur if adequately excised.

Calcinosis circumscripta *(Fig.* 2.14)

This lesion is seen most commonly in young dogs of the large breeds, particularly Irish Wolfhounds and Alsatians. It consists of a firm irregular mass or masses in the dermis over the limb joints, the dorsal aspect of the neck and sometimes in the tongue. The lesions have a characteristic appearance on the cut surface. They are composed of irregular chalky white foci separated by grey–white fibrous tissue. Radiologically and histologically these foci are seen to be heavily calcified. The cause of calcinosis circumscripta is not known but the marked breed incidence suggests there may be a genetic influence in its development.

Treatment. Excision is the treatment of choice.

Lick granuloma *(Fig.* 2.15)

This lesion occurs predominantly in the larger breeds such as Labradors, Retrievers, Dobermans and Great Danes. It is caused by persistent licking and biting, probably as the result of boredom. The lesions occur most commonly on the anterior carpal or metacarpal region but also can arise on the anterior aspect of the more proximal regions of fore and hind limbs. They are thickened, firm, ulcerated lesions which often have a hyperpigmented halo in the more chronic stages of their development.

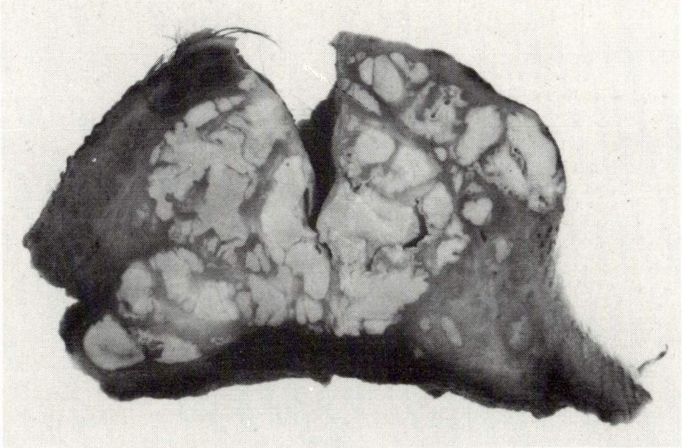

Fig. 2.14. Calcinosis circumscripta adjacent to the dew claw of a 10-month-old Irish Wolfhound. Similar lesions were present along the edge of this dog's tongue.

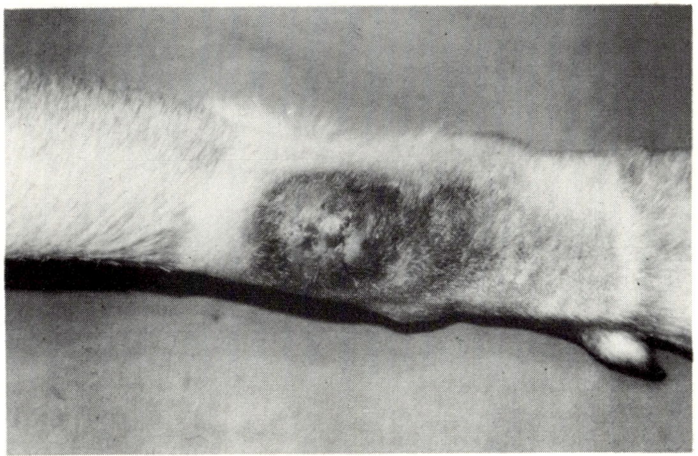

Fig. 2.15. Carpal lick granuloma on an 8-year-old Labrador dog.

Treatment. If the licking habit cannot be broken in some way then the prognosis should be guarded since, even after excision of the original lesion, the dog may produce further granulomas. Injection of corticosteroid into the granuloma is said to be useful in the treatment of early lesions.

REFERENCES

Bostock D. E. (1973) The prognosis following surgical removal of mastocytomas in dogs. *J. Small. Anim. Pract.* **14**, 27–40.

Bostock D. E. and Owen L. N. (1975) *A Colour Atlas of Neoplasia in the Cat, Dog and Horse.* London, Wolfe Medical.

Brodey R. S. (1970) Canine and feline neoplasia. *Adv. Vet. Sci.* **14**, 309–54.

Cotchin E. (1961) Skin tumours of cats. *Res. Vet. Sci.* **2**, 353–61.

Dorn C. R., Taylor D. O. N., Schneider R. et al. (1968) Survey of animal neoplasms in Alameda and Contra Costa counties, California. II. Cancer morbidity in dogs and cats from Alameda county. *J. Natl Cancer Inst.* **40**, 307–18.

Mc Chesney A. E., Stephens J. L., Snyder S. et al. (1980) Infiltrative lipoma in dogs. *Vet. Path.* **17**, 316–22.

Moulton J. E. (1978) *Tumours in Domestic Animals,* 2nd ed. Berkeley, Ca, University of California Press.

Priester W. A. (1973) Skin tumors in domestic animals. Data from 12 United States and Canadian Colleges of Veterinary Medicine. *J. Natl Cancer Inst.* **50**, 457–66.

Priester W. A. and Mantel N. (1971) Occurrence of tumours in domestic animals. Data from 12 United States and Canadian Colleges of Veterinary Medicine. *J. Natl Cancer Inst.* **47**, 1333–44.

Schneider R. (1975) A population based animal tumour registry. In: Ingram D.G., Mitchell W. R. and Martin S. W. (ed.) *Animal Disease Monitoring.* Springfield, Ill, Thomas.

Wilkinson G. T., Kelly W. R. and O'Boyle D. (1978) Cutaneous granulomas associated with *Mycobacterium fortuitum* in a cat. *J. Small Anim. Pract.* **19**, 357–62.

Chapter 3

Surgical Pathology

II: The Mammary Glands

Mammary tumours in the dog are second in frequency only to those of the skin and in the bitch they are the commonest of all spontaneous neoplasms. In the cat mammary tumours are not as common, accounting for less than 10 per cent of all tumours (Priester and Mantel, 1971). They are, however, more predictable and constant in their behaviour than mammary tumours in the bitch. More than 80 per cent of feline mammary tumours are malignant. Most are adenocarcinomas that grow rapidly causing ulceration, local infiltration and early metastasis to drainage lymph nodes and to the lungs. In contrast, probably less than 50 per cent of mammary tumours in the bitch are malignant and there is still controversy and confusion amongst pathologists about the nomenclature and histogenesis of these tumours.

Aetiology

There are many unfounded statements about the aetiology of mammary neoplasia, particularly in the dog. Such statements relate especially to the influence of endocrine factors on the incidence and behaviour of mammary tumours. In the past decade certain facts have emerged which are well-supported by carefully analysed data, although the precise hormonal or other influences in the development of mammary neoplasia have yet to be clarified.

The following general statements about the influence of hormonal factors on mammary neoplasia in the bitch can be made.

1. There is no evidence of an increased incidence of mammary neoplasia in bitches with irregularities of the oestrus cycle, or in those that have never bred. Age- and breed-matched control bitches without mammary tumours show the same frequency of abnormalities of the oestrus cycle

and breeding pattern as do those with tumours (Brodey et al., 1966). There is conflicting evidence, however, on the association between unusually severe pseudopregnancies and mammary neoplasia. Brodey and his colleagues (1966) stated that there is no relationship between the two. More recently Else and Hannant (1979) have shown that bitches with marked pseudopregnancies have a significantly increased incidence of mammary tumours.

2. Bitches spayed before 2 years of age have a greatly reduced risk of developing mammary neoplasia later in life. This sparing effect does not operate if spaying is delayed until the bitch is 2½ years old or later.

3. Ovariectomy does not cause regression of already established tumours or their metastases.

Hormonal factors in the development of mammary neoplasia

There is now a considerable body of information on the influence of various hormonal factors on the development and treatment of breast cancer in women. It is now possible to detect specific receptor proteins in tumour cells which bind steroid hormones in the cytoplasm or nucleus of the cell. Such methods make it possible to identify those tumours which are hormone-dependent and which are likely, therefore, to respond to anti-hormone treatment or to endocrine ablation.

The study of hormone receptor sites in canine and feline mammary neoplasia is still in its infancy. Even if it becomes easy to demonstrate that some tumours are hormone-dependent it is debatable whether endocrine ablation, as practised in human medicine, would be feasible or desirable. Information on hormones which may influence the development or behaviour of mammary tumours in the dog and cat is discussed briefly below.

Oestrogens and progestagens

Oestrogens are known to be essential factors for both the induction and maintenance of experimental mammary carcinomas in some laboratory animals. In women, some breast cancers are oestrogen-dependent and anti-hormone therapy or endocrine ablation can be useful in the treatment of inoperable tumours and of metastatic disease. There is considerable debate, however, as to whether the prolonged use of oestrogenic drugs increases the risk of breast cancer in women.

Prolonged use of various synthetic oestrogens in Beagle bitches does not appear to cause any increase in the development of mammary tumours, although they do produce other tumours.

Recently, oestrogen receptors have been demonstrated in spontaneous canine mammary tumours and in a small number of feline mammary carcinomas but considerably more work is required to determine what proportion of tumours in these species bear oestrogen receptors.

At the time of writing no work appears to have been done to demonstrate the presence of other hormone receptors in either canine or feline mammary tumours. This is surprising in view of the fact that there is now a considerable volume of literature showing that long-term dosing with certain synthetic progestagens causes an increased incidence of mammary tumours in Beagle bitches. Furthermore, the occasional occurrence of mammary carcinomas in cats given prolonged progestagen treatment suggests that these hormones may be important also in the pathogenesis of feline mammary neoplasia, but experimental proof is lacking at present.

Pituitary and other hormones

Recent work suggests that growth hormone in the dog plays an important role in the pathogenesis of spontaneous and progestagen-related mammary tumours. Investigations on prolactin, which has been incriminated as a maintenance factor in human breast cancer, suggest that it is not involved in experimental or spontaneous neoplasia in the dog. Similar information is not available for feline mammary carcinoma and data on the influence of other pituitary, adrenal and thyroid hormones in the dog at present are limited and confusing.

Viruses and mammary neoplasia

Virus-like particles have been detected by electron microscopy in some feline mammary carcinomas. Both C-type and A-type particles have been identified in approximately 25 per cent of a small group of feline mammary carcinomas. They were not found in benign tumours nor in normal mammary glands. However, it has not been possible so far to induce mammary neoplasia by the injection of cell-free homogenates of virus-containing neoplasms into new-born kittens. Until this can be done there is no proof that viruses can induce mammary neoplasia in the cat.

Viruses do not appear to have been implicated as a cause of mammary neoplasia in the bitch.

Summary

Oestrogens

1. Prolonged administration of several types of synthetic oestrogens in Beagles does not increase the incidence of mammary tumours.

2. Oestrogen receptors have been demonstrated in some spontaneous canine and feline tumours. Information is lacking on the proportion of tumours bearing such receptors and on the influence of anti-hormone therapy or endocrine ablation on established hormone-dependent tumours.

Progestagens

1. Long term experimental use of several different progestagens causes an increased incidence of mammary tumours in Beagle bitches.

2. There are reports of mammary carcinomas developing in cats on prolonged progestagen therapy. This may be purely coincidental and these observations require experimental corroboration.

Pituitary hormones

1. Present evidence suggests that growth hormone, but not prolactin, may be important in the pathogenesis of spontaneous and progestagen-induced canine mammary tumours.

2. Information is lacking or confusing on the role of other hormones from the pituitary, adrenal and thyroid in the pathogenesis of mammary neoplasia in the dog and cat.

Viruses

1. Although virus-like particles have been seen in some feline mammary carcinomas, proof is lacking that they are the cause of the tumours.

2. Viruses have not been implicated as a cause of mammary neoplasia in the bitch.

MAMMARY NEOPLASIA IN THE CAT

This is an important group of tumours in the cat because, although not as common as in the dog, a very much higher percentage of them are malignant (over 80 per cent). Most are well-differentiated adenocarcinomas, mesenchymal and mixed tumours being very rare in the cat.

There is strong evidence that early spaying markedly reduces the incidence of mammary neoplasia in later life, as it does in the bitch.

Age

Most tumours occur in old cats (average 12½ years) (Brodey, 1970), although the author has seen aggressive adenocarcinomas in a few cats less than 3 years old.

Sites and gross appearance

All four glands appear to be equally susceptible to tumour formation. The tumours at first may appear well demarcated and benign but more often they are already fixed to underlying tissues and may even be ulcerated when first presented. Infiltration of local lymphatics may cause oedematous thickening of the surrounding skin. They are usually firm nodular tumours, poorly demarcated and infiltrative.

Behaviour and treatment

In most cases of feline mammary neoplasia the prognosis is very poor. The tumours commonly recur after removal. They grow rapidly and tend to metastasize early to local lymph nodes and to the lungs. Some invade through the thoracic wall and produce pleural metastases.

Feline mammary hypertrophy

This is an uncommon non-neoplastic lesion of the mammary glands of the cat. It occurs in adolescent female cats, young pregnant and non-pregnant queens and occasionally in neutered male and female cats receiving prolonged doses of the progestagen, megoestrol acetate.

Site and gross appearance

One, several or all the glands may be involved, with firm, painless swellings. The swelling often causes such gross enlargement of the glands that the overlying skin is stretched and ulcerated. In neutered cats receiving megoestrol acetate the lesions are more localized, sometimes cystic, and usually involve only one or two of the glands.

Microscopic appearances

The lesions are composed of lobules of proliferating ducts surrounded by active oedematous and cellular connective tissue. The interlobular septa are more collagenous and less cellular than the stroma surrounding the ducts.

Behaviour and treatment

The masses often develop at an alarming rate, particularly in the young pregnant and non-pregnant queens. A much lower rate of growth occurs in the cats receiving hormone therapy.

Softening and gradual regression of the lesions over 6–8 weeks follows ovariohysterectomy in the young queens. Treatment of the more localized lesions seen in the neutered cats receiving hormone therapy consists of surgical excision of the lesion and withdrawal or reduction of the dosage of megoestrol acetate.

Aetiology

It seems likely that the cause of this unusual condition in the cat is either an exaggerated and idiosyncratic response of the mammary gland to normal progesterone levels or that it is the result of increased progesterone levels.

MAMMARY NEOPLASIA IN THE BITCH

Mammary tumours are the most common group of tumours in the bitch and represent a significant proportion of the surgical cases seen in small animal practice. Some of the misconceptions and confusion which have arisen over the relationship between hormonal disturbances and mammary neoplasia have already been dealt with in the early part of this chapter.

There still remains, however, considerable debate and confusion amongst pathologists about the histogenesis and methods of classifying canine mammary tumours. This arises because of the extremely variable histological appearance they display. A large proportion of the tumours (approximately 60 per cent) contain both epithelial and mesenchymal elements such as myxomatous tissue, cartilage, osteoid and bone. Such tumours have been called 'complex' or 'mixed' mammary tumours on the assumption that both the epithelial and mesenchymal components have undergone neoplastic change. A recent careful study from the Tulsa Registry of Canine and Feline Neoplasms (Monlux et al., 1977) casts considerable doubt on this assumption. Their findings strongly suggest that the mesenchymal components in mixed mammary tumours are metaplastic changes with no neoplastic potential and that they occur in response to leakage into the stroma of secretions from the neoplastic epithelial cells. Their classification of canine mammary tumours is, therefore, very much less complex than that, for example, of the World Health Organisation, and it is outlined below:

Benign mammary tumours	Adenoma Ductal papilloma	approximately equal in frequency
Malignant mammary tumours	Ductal carcinoma	by far the most common
	Lobular carcinoma Squamous cell carcinoma	both rare

It may be that this classification of canine mammary tumours will be adopted by pathologists in the future and that the terms 'mixed' or 'complex' mammary tumours will disappear from our reports. I suspect, however, that there always will be some who continue to use these terms even though present evidence suggests that they are incorrect.

Age

The incidence of mammary tumours begins to increase rapidly at about 6 years of age and is said to decrease after 11 years of age.

Sites and gross appearances

There is a much greater frequency of tumour development in the two most caudal glands than in the anterior glands. Both benign and malignant neoplasms occur more frequently at this site and there appears to be no support for the belief that tumours in the anterior glands are most likely to be malignant.

Benign tumours are usually freely movable beneath the skin and over the underlying tissues, although the larger tumours may become traumatically ulcerated. They feel well-circumscribed and usually shell out easily at surgery. They may be rounded, nodular, solid or cystic. If cartilage or bone is present in significant amounts it often can be detected when the tumour is incised.

Malignant tumours become fixed to the underlying tissues by infiltration, and invasion of the overlying skin causes a dimpled orange-peel effect followed by ulceration. They are difficult to delineate and will invade adjacent glands. Infiltration of local dermal lymphatics may cause obstruction to lymphatic drainage which results in gross thickening of the skin and hind limb oedema. Occasionally a very aggressive form of carcinoma develops simultaneously in all mammary glands and may be mistaken for mastitis.

Drainage lymph nodes should always be examined for evidence of metastases and submitted together with the tumour to the pathologist. The two anterior glands drain into the axillary lymph node while the caudal two glands drain to the inguinal lymph node. The middle gland (gland 3) usually drains to both nodes. When tumours are removed from the fifth gland the inguinal lymph node is nearly always removed with them. It is rare, however, for the axillary gland to be removed unless it is very obviously enlarged.

Behaviour and treatment

Benign tumours, which account for 50–60 per cent of all mammary tumours, grow slowly, often over a very long period. They may, however, show an increase in size immediately after oestrus and it is important that the date of the last heat is always noted on the form submitted to the pathologist. Clinically benign tumours should be removed by simple mastectomy as soon as possible. When tumours are multiple it may be necessary to remove the whole or part of the mammary gland chain on one or both sides.

Malignant tumours usually grow rapidly and this rapidity of growth is probably the most useful factor in their clinical assessment. Some, however, may have a history of slow growth for months, followed by a sudden increase in size. Suggestions that there is positive correlation between the size of malignant tumours and their prognosis appear to be misleading. It is not known what proportion of benign tumours, if left, will later become malignant and for this reason it is important that all mammary tumours should be removed, as soon as possible after they are first recognized. Monlux and his colleagues (1977) believe that all carcinomas begin as benign growths but that most become malignant within a few weeks of their inception. Their findings suggest that if ductal carcinomas are removed when they are showing early histological evidence of invasion then the prognosis is good. Tumours that show greater degrees of invasion generally carry a poor prognosis. They recur and will metastasize to local lymph nodes and to the lungs, often in less than 1 year after surgery. Recent surveys indicate that a high proportion of dogs with carcinomas have died or are killed as a direct result of their tumours within 2 years of surgery: Bostock (1975), 43 per cent; Misdorp and Hart (1976), 75 per cent; Else and Hannant (1979), 60 per cent.

Radical mastectomy is the treatment of choice but it may be difficult to delineate aggressive, highly invasive tumours. Some of the rapidly growing carcinomas respond to X-irradiation but in most cases it appears to be of little value. In spite of this it is sometimes surprising to find bitches surviving for many months even when pulmonary metastases have been recognized.

NON-NEOPLASTIC TUMOUR-LIKE LESIONS OF THE MAMMARY GLAND IN THE BITCH

Several types of non-neoplastic lesion are found in the dog's mammary gland. Some arise in association with the changes of proliferation and involution that occur during the oestrus cycle, others occur independent of these cyclical changes.

Normally during metoestrus there is proliferation of ductular and acinar tissue until about 6 weeks after oestrus when involution starts to occur in the non-pregnant bitch. Secretion is evident in alveoli at the time of maximum lobular development and this secretory activity is exaggerated in bitches that are pseudopregnant.

Cystic hyperplasia (Mammary dysplasia, cystic mastopathy)

The mammary glands do not always respond uniformly throughout to successive hormonal cycles. Some lobules may not undergo the normal cyclical regression outlined above and eventually they form palpable nodules indistinguishable clinically from neoplastic nodules. Microscopically they present a variety of morphological appearances that may be difficult to differentiate from benign tumours. Inflammatory changes may be superimposed on hyperplastic lesions.

Duct ectasia

This change, as its name implies, is one of marked dilatation of ducts
and ductules. It may occur in cystic hyperplastic nodules or it may arise
on its own. The nodules have a soft spongy appearance and in the most
severe cases the entire gland may be replaced by a spongy mass. Inflammatory changes may be superimposed on those of duct ectasia, particularly when ducts rupture, releasing their contents into the surrounding
stroma.

Fat necrosis

This is not a common lesion in the mammary gland but it may arise in
obese bitches and is probably the result of trauma. Foci of fat necrosis
present as firm discrete masses in the gland, which have an opaque yellow-
white appearance often mottled by haemorrhagic areas. The lesion is
always associated with varying degrees of inflammation.

Mastitis

Although normally a condition that arises during early lactation, mastitis
can occur at other stages of the oestrus cycle, particularly during pseudo-
pregnancy. Foci of mastitis may be mistaken for neoplasms when they
occur outside the lactation period.

REFERENCES

Bostock D. E. (1975) The prognosis following surgical excision of canine mammary
    neoplasms. *Eur. J. Cancer* **11,** 389–96.
Brodey R. S. (1970) Canine and feline neoplasia. *Adv. Vet. Sci.* **14,** 309–54.
Brodey R. S., Fidler I. J. and Howson A. E. (1966) The relationship of estrus irregu-
    larities, pseudopregnancy and pregnancy to the development of canine mammary
    neoplasms. *J. Am. Vet. Med. Assoc.* **149,** 1047–9.
Else R. W. and Hannant D. (1979) Some epidemiological aspects of mammary
    neoplasia in the bitch. *Vet. Rec.* **104,** 296–304.
Misdorp W. and Hart A. A. M. (1976) Prognostic factors in canine mammary cancer.
    J. Natl Cancer Inst. **56,** 779–86.
Monlux A. W., Roszel J. F., McVean D. W. et al. (1977) Classification of epithelial
    canine mammary tumours in a defined population. *Vet. Path.* **14,** 194–217.
Priester W. A. and Mantel N. (1971) Occurrence of tumours in domestic animals.
    Data from 12 United States and Canadian Colleges of Veterinary Medicine.
    J. Natl Cancer Inst. **47,** 1333–44.

Chapter 4

Necropsy Procedures

For the small animal practitioner the principal reasons for carrying out
necropsies (Gk *nekros* – corpse) are to confirm or refute a clinical diagnosis
or impression, to define more precisely the type and extent of lesions
causing clinical disease, or to establish the cause of death. In some situations the objective of the necropsy may be quite limited, and this may be
achieved by a partial post-mortem examination. For example, the presence
of diaphragmatic rupture or pleural empyema can be confirmed on visual
examination of the opened thorax. Many illnesses, however, are less simple
and proper necropsy demands that the carcass be examined fully so that a
complete assessment of the state of the tissues can be obtained. To do this
requires a thorough systematic approach so that the main body systems
are examined and all deviations from normal recorded. The need for a
systematic approach is not mere pedantry: practice in the methods outlined here ensures that time is not wasted on random fumbling or
unnecessarily intricate dissection!

The following approach is recommended as one found useful by the
author but it can be modified as necessary to conform with the specific
requirements of the clinician, or with the limitations imposed by practice
conditions.

APPROACH TO THE NECROPSY

Clinical history and examination

The practitioner who autopsies his own former patients will generally have
all the details of history, clinical and laboratory examinations, treatments
and clinical course. If this is not the case it is important to review this
information as fully as possible: this may provide a clinical diagnosis of

varying firmness and may indicate the need to examine particular organs with special care. Occasionally the clinical history may suggest the need for special tissue fixatives.

Wherever possible the animal should be weighed before opening the carcass. This provides an objective measurement of body size and is essential if relative organ weights are to be assessed.

External examination

The next stage involves a systematic examination to look for evidence of trauma, recent surgery, anaemic mucous membranes or jaundice. At the same time an assessment can be made of body condition. A check-list of the features to be noted in an external examination is shown in Table 4.1.

Post-mortem instruments

These should be reserved exclusively for necropsy work and should be cleaned and autoclaved or soaked in disinfectant after use. The principal requirement is for a stout butcher's knife: this is used for making most of the incisions and needs to be kept sharp with a wet stone and butcher's steel. Surgical scalpels should not be substituted for a stout knife: the

Table 4.1. Check-list for external examination of small animal carcasses prior to necropsy

Head	Buccal and conjunctival mucous membranes: examine for evidence of anaemia, haemorrhage, jaundice
	Examine for: Congenital abnormalities (cleft palate)
	Teeth – dental wear
	– dental calculi
	– paradontal disease
Neck	Palpate submaxillary and prescapular lymph nodes
Forelimbs	Examine for venepuncture marks
	Wear on claws, tearing of claws (trauma)
	Palpation for evidence of trauma
Thorax	Palpation for evidence of trauma
Abdomen	Palpation for evidence of abdominal enlargement due to fluid accumulation
	Palpation of mammary glands for evidence of nodularity, secretion
	Examination of prepuce – preputial discharge
	Palpation of testes for evidence of enlargement, nodularity, cryptorchidism
	Examination of anus – diarrhoea, perianal gland nodularity, perianal ulceration
Hind limbs	Palpation for evidence of trauma

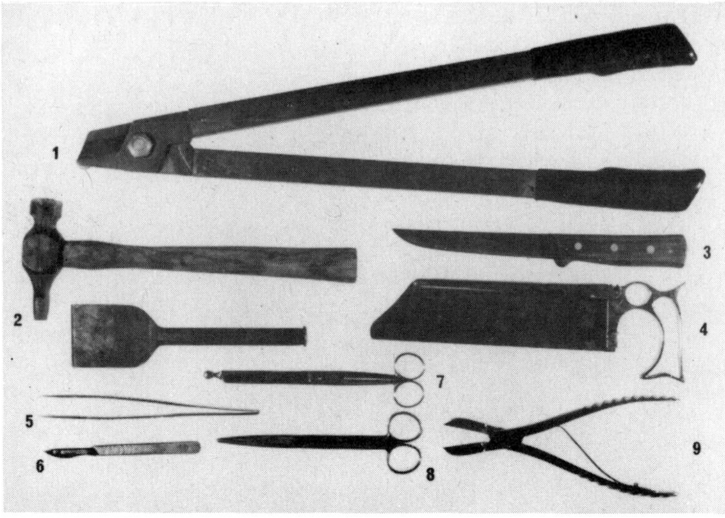

Fig. 4.1. Set of instruments for small animal post-mortem work **1**, Rib shears. **2**, Hammer and chisel (skull removal). **3**, Butcher's knife. **4**, Bone saw. **5**, Rat-tooth forceps. **6**, Scalpel (for fine dissection). **7**, Bowel scissors. **8**, Round-ended dissecting scissors. **9**, Bone forceps.

blades frequently break, they rapidly become blunt and accidents are more likely to result from their use. A suitable range of necropsy instruments is illustrated in *Fig.* 4.1.

NECROPSY PROCEDURES

Primary incision

The animal is placed on its back and deep incisions made in the axillae and groins. A long mid-line ventral incision is made through the skin from the mandibular symphysis to the pubic brim. In the male dog it is convenient to incise along both sides of the prepuce so that the penis can be reflected in a caudal direction. The skin is now reflected from the lateral aspects of the neck, thorax, abdomen and thighs (*Fig.* 4.2). At this stage the exposed subcutaneous tissues are examined for the presence of anaemia or haemorrhage, congestion, jaundice, adipose tissue. When laparotomy has been carried out the incision should be examined for the presence of oedema, haemorrhage, wound breakdown or infection. Before opening the body cavities the superficial lymph nodes (submaxillary, prescapular) are located, palpated and multiple incisions made through their capsules. The normal prescapular nodes are usually small and difficult to locate, especially in the obese subject: if multiple incisions through the prescapular regions

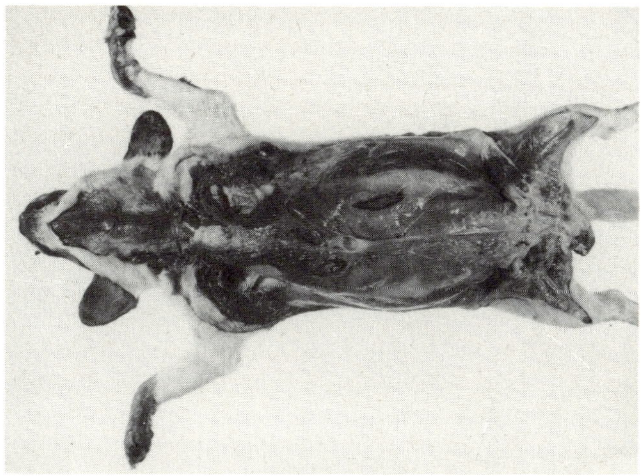

Fig. 4.2. Primary incision with ventral skin reflected from the angle of the jaw
to the pubis and thighs.

fail to reveal the lymph nodes it can be assumed that they are not enlarged.
Multiple incisions are made through the mammary tissue on both sides,
noting the location, size and consistency of any abnormal areas.

Exposure of body cavities

A small incision is made in the umbilical region and this is extended gently
in cranial and caudal directions. The state of the exposed peritoneum is
examined and if abnormal peritoneal fluid is present it can be collected
and measured. The normal peritoneum in dogs and cats is smooth, glistening and transparent and the abdominal cavity normally contains only a
few millilitres of clear, colourless, unclotted fluid. If excess fluid is present
a small aliquot is withdrawn into a sterile syringe for subsequent microbiological, biochemical or cytological examination. The abdominal cavity
is now opened by making deep ventrodorsal incisions through the lateral
abdominal walls.

The abdominal viscera are examined *in situ,* noting any abnormalities in
position or alterations in size. The thorax is opened by cutting through the
left side of the chest approximately midway between the sternum and the
head of the ribs, using rib shears (*Fig.* 4.1). The cut edge of the thoracic
wall is now lifted and reflected, exposing the thoracic cavity and contents
(*Fig.* 4.3). At this stage it is convenient to examine the pleural cavities for
the presence of fluid. If excess fluid is present a small aliquot is withdrawn
into a sterile syringe for subsequent microbiological, biochemical or
cytological examination. Residual fluid is collected and measured. The

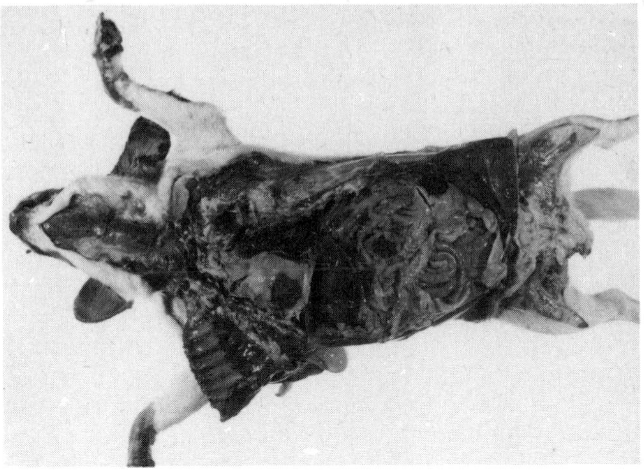

Fig. 4.3. Exposure of abdominal and thoracic cavities.

normal canine and feline pleura is smooth, glistening and transparent and the pleural cavities normally contain a few millilitres of clear, colourless, unclotted fluid.

The sternum is now reflected towards the right side and the ventral mediastinal tissues freed from the parietal pleura. A longitudinal incision is made through the costochondral junctions on the right side and the ventral wall of the thorax can be freed easily, cutting through the intercostal muscles with a knife. A routine procedure at this stage is to make deep incisions through the intercostal muscles and attempt to fracture several ribs with the hands. Experience of the normal strength and consistency of rib bone is useful in assessing pathological fragility in nutritional and renal osteodystrophies. Bone strength varies considerably in normal animals, depending on body size. It is convenient at this stage to open the shoulder, hips and stifle joint cavities, and to inspect articular cartilage and synovium.

Examination of organ systems

Alimentary tract

It is convenient to first remove the spleen and omentum. The colon is now located and a transverse incision made cranial to the pubic brim. With the incised lower end of the colon held in the left hand, the mesentery is cut with scissors and the incision continued forward to the lower end of the duodenum. The mesenteric incision should be as close to the viscera as possible — this allows the intestines to be opened rapidly. If a long length of mesentery is left attached to the intestines, opening of the bowel is made much more tedious. The duodenum is transected and the small and large intestines removed from the abdomen.

If quantitative parasitological examination of the bowel lumina is contemplated the small and large intestines are first ligated with string or other suitable material before being transected. The bowel is examined and palpated and then opened along the anti-mesenteric aspect using bowel scissors, noting the appearance of the mucosa, the quality of the contents, the presence of inflamed or ulcerated mucosa and the presence of round-worms or tapeworms. Gentle washing of the mucosa of the large bowel may be necessary to remove adherent contents. The normal mucosa of the small intestine is turgid and thick in the live animal or immediately post mortem. After death autolytic changes result in detachment of mucosa so that the bowel wall becomes correspondingly thinner. Regional variation in apparent vascularity of the small intestinal mucosa is common in the dog and cat; this may become more apparent when post-mortem autolytic thinning occurs and has to be distinguished from active inflammatory hyperaemia or passive congestion of the bowel.

The stomach, duodenum, liver and pancreas are now removed *in toto:* the ventral edge of the diaphragm is held in the left hand and a wide incision is made around the edge of the diaphragm close to its lateral attachments. At this stage care is taken to avoid tearing or incising the right adrenal gland which is closely attached to the posterior edge of the liver and the posterior vena cava (*see below*).

The liver surface is examined for evidence of nodules, adhesions, fibrous plaques or tears. The gallbladder is palpated to test (albeit crudely) for patency of the bile ducts. Bile can be expressed easily into the duo-denum by gentle pressure on the gallbladder. Mild obstruction of the extrahepatic biliary tract cannot be appreciated by palpation but occasion-ally gross obstruction of the bile ducts (by calculi) is seen — obstruction of this severity can be appreciated by the failure of manual emptying of the gallbladder. Passage of bile into the duodenum can usually be appreciated by swelling in the ampullary region or after incision along the anti-mesenteric border of the duodenum. The gallbladder is opened along its length with scissors; dissection of the major bile ducts in dogs and cats requires small dissecting scissors and a degree of patience that is rarely rewarded by the demonstration of significant lesions. The normal mucosa of the gallbladder is smooth, green and mucoid; the contents are usually dark green and often contain soft, dark green floccular material. Multiple transverse incisions are made through the liver substance. In the dog the cut surfaces are usually uniformly dark; in the cat a lobular pattern is more distinct and relative pallor is a normal feature.

The stomach and duodenum are opened along the anti-mesenteric border to expose the mucosa. In the dog the gastric rugal folds are well developed and the duodenal mucosa is often normally red and variably stained with bile. Post-prandial hyperaemia of the gastric mucosa is a

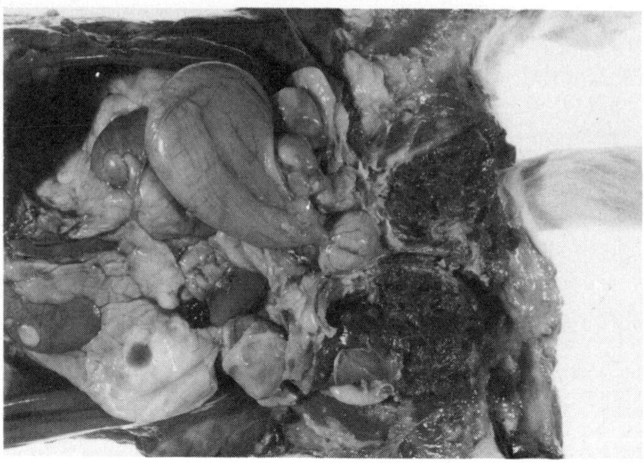

Fig. 4.4. The ventromedial part of the pelvis has been removed, exposing the urethra and allowing the lower urogenital tract, rectum and anus to be removed together.

normal physiological response and, if there is food in the stomach, should not be confused with pathological hyperaemia. The duodenal and mesenteric limbs of the pancreas are palpated and incised: in both dog and cat this gland is pale cream-pink and distinctly lobulated.

The mesentery and mesenteric lymph nodes are removed finally. The terminal colon, rectum and anus are examined later, together with the urogenital organs.

Urogenital system

It is helpful to maintain the anatomical relationships of the urogenital system and this is achieved by first removing the floor of the pelvis. Parallel cuts are made with rib shears through the pubic brim into the obturator foramina and through the ischia. The medial part of the pelvis is removed (*Fig.* 4.4). A knife is used to cut around the anus and the adjacent vulva or penis. The lower urogenital organs, the rectum and anus can now be pulled away from the pelvis. The kidneys and ovaries are palpated for any abnormality before the lower urogenital organs are lifted in a cranial direction, tearing the peritoneal attachments and reflections from the ovaries, uterine horns and kidneys.

Systematic examination of the urogenital tract follows. The kidneys are sliced longitudinally along a horizontal plane from the capsule to the hilus. The capsules are pulled away from the cortical surface. In the normal canine kidney there are usually no more than occasional fibrous connections of the capsule to the cortex. The consistency of the renal cut surfaces is noted; there is usually moderately clear demarcation of the cortex from the paler medulla. Radial striation is a normal feature in the latter. The renal pelvic cavities are opened fully with scissors to expose the fornices. Complete dissection of the ureters is tedious and requires the use of fine dissecting scissors. Random transverse slicing of the kidneys is carried out to look for focal lesions not revealed by the primary incision.

The urinary bladder is palpated before being incised with scissors in the fundic region. The incision is continued in a posterior direction into the urethra and through the lower urinary tract. The mucosa of the urethra is normally dark due to the underlying venous plexuses. In the male the prostate is palpated and then sliced transversely at intervals of a few millimetres. Complete dissection of the male urethra requires fine scissors to pass through the os penis. The prepuce is opened throughout its length. The scrotum is incised carefully to expose the testes, epididymis and spermatic cords; the testes are palpated to detect focal lesions. Slicing of the unfixed testes produces artefacts in subsequent tissue sections so it is preferable to fix the gonads for a few days before systematic examination.

Examination of the female genitalia involves complete opening of the tubular organs from the vulva to the cranial extremities of the uterine horns. This is usually done with large dissecting scissors, although a finer pair is necessary to open the cervix. The ovaries are exposed by opening the ovarian bursae and reflecting the fatty wall. The ovaries are examined for follicles and corpora lutea by palpation and slicing.

Respiratory system

After opening the thorax and inspecting the pleura the prosector grasps and cuts the aorta and oesophagus immediately cranial to the diaphragm. The thoracic organs can then be pulled in a cranial direction and removed from the chest. The heart, lungs and trachea can be pulled and cut from the ventral muscles of the neck. The hyoid bones are cut with bone forceps or stout scissors and the tongue and pharynx freed by cutting. The tongue is pulled ventrally from the mouth and the cardiorespiratory organs removed from the carcass.

The organs are rested in their natural position on a suitable surface for dissection and the dorsal wall of the pharynx incised longitudinally with scissors. The tongue, pharnyx and tonsils are thereby fully exposed for inspection, palpation and slicing. The oesophagus is opened along its length and then pulled away from the underlying trachea. Separation of the organs in this way exposes the thyroid glands which are situated lateral to the trachea immediately posterior to the larynx. The thyroids are small pink-red structures measuring up to 2 cm in length and up to 0·5 cm in diameter; the parathyroids are smaller cream-white organs that often bulge from the lateral aspect of the thyroids, although there is considerable variation between individuals in the thyroid/parathyroid relationship.

Further examination of the respiratory tract is preceded by careful palpation of the lung lobes. Small foci of consolidation may be recognized more readily by palpation than by dissection since the fingers can easily appreciate the contrast between aerated and consolidated lung. Complete exposure of the airway conducting system is produced by longitudinal opening of the larynx, trachea and bronchi. In older dogs the bronchial cartilages are often calcified or ossified, producing a gritty sensation as the rings are cut. The mucosa of the conducting airways is normally smooth, glistening and pale.

Inspection of the nasal chambers and paranasal sinuses is carried out by incision and reflection of the nasal skin and by opening the cavities with bone saws and forceps. The normal mucosa of the nasal turbinates is smooth, glistening and red. This results from the normal vascularity and should not be mistaken for pathological hyperaemia. Mucosa of the nasal sinuses is smooth, glistening and pale.

Cardiovascular system

The lungs and heart are rested on a dissecting surface with the heart uppermost. The pericardial sac is palpated for evidence of abnormal fluid accumulation. The sac normally contains a few millilitres of clear, colourless, unclotted fluid. Excess fluid can be aspirated through the sac into a syringe for cytological or biochemical examination: if microbiological examination is expected the pericardial sac should first be sterilized by searing with a spatula, iron or scalpel blade heated in a bunsen burner. The pericardial sac is now opened with scissors from the apex to the base of the heart and the epicardium inspected. The epicardium is normally smooth and glistening.

Opening and dissection of the heart should follow a logical sequence but the incisions should not be so numerous that the heart cannot be reconstructed for demonstration. Several methods of dissection are practised; the following is a simple one based on the normal blood flow through the heart. The anterior and posterior venae cavae are incised longitudinally with scissors and post-mortem blood clot removed. The right atrium is exposed by a longitudinal cut towards the auricular tip. Post-mortem blood clot is frequently found in the atria and gentle traction may be necessary to detach this from the endocardial surfaces. The tricuspid valve orifice is inspected for normal patency, valvular thickening or endocarditis. The right ventricle is then opened with scissors, cutting through the tricuspid valve, continuing towards the apex and then turning dorsally towards the pulmonary valve and into the main pulmonary arterial trunk. The incision that opens the right side of the heart is made as close as possible to the interventricular septum (*Fig.* 4.5). The left

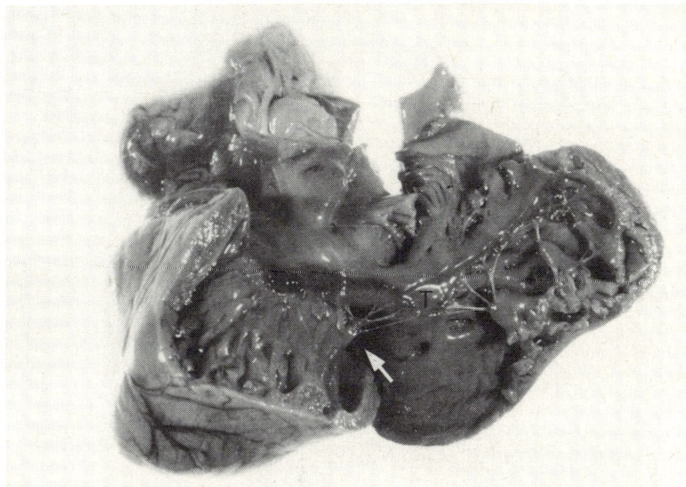

Fig. 4.5. Canine heart with right side exposed revealing tricuspid valve (T) and pulmonary outflow (arrow).

side of the heart is opened in a similar manner, beginning in the pulmonary veins and finishing by opening the aortic trunk (*Fig.* 4.6). At this last point the prosector will have to cut across the root of the opened pulmonary artery. The valves are examined systematically and multiple transverse incisions are made into the myocardium of the lateral walls of the ventricles

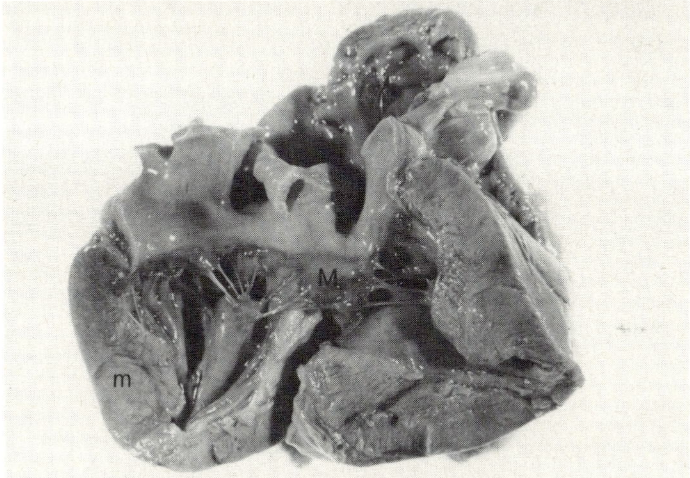

Fig. 4.6. Canine heart with left side exposed revealing mitral valve (M), papillary muscle and ventricular myocardium (m).

and of the interventricular septum. Experience in carrying out necropsies on dogs and cats will provide subjective appreciation of the normal thickness of the myocardium. Gross hypertrophy and dilatation can be readily appreciated but less severe adaptive changes may present difficulties in assessment. The coronary arteries can be dissected from their ostia using fine-pointed scissors. The large extramural coronary arteries are only rarely the site of disease in the dog and detailed dissection is rarely rewarding, except to confirm the absence of lesions.

Lymphoreticular system

The spleen is examined by palpation and transverse slicing. In young animals the Malpighian follicles are normally conspicuous, appearing as white nodules of up to 1–2 mm in diameter. Random slices are made through the mesenteric, sternal, bronchial and iliac lymph nodes. The lymph nodes are normally larger in the young animal and have firm, pale and conspicuously follicular cut surfaces. Bone-marrow can be examined in a longitudinal slice of sternum, or from the medulla of the femur. In the puppy and kitten active red marrow is present throughout the length of the long bone shafts, but in the adult the haemopoietic tissue is confined to the metaphyseal regions. Some indication of the relative cellularity of the marrow can be gained by immersion of the tissue in fixative: active red marrow will sink, whereas marrow with a large proportion of adipose tissue will float.

Endocrine system

Examination of the endocrine glands should be limited to noting any gross abnormality of size. Thyroids and pituitary (*see below*) can be fixed whole in formalin. The adrenals should be carefully dissected from surrounding fat before being fixed whole. Attempts to cut unfixed endocrine glands usually result in crushing; furthermore there are relatively few clinical diseases in which confident pathological diagnosis can be made on the naked eye appearances, so it is preferable to obtain optimally fixed material for histological examination. The adrenal cortex has a distinct yellow–cream appearance, due to its high lipid content, and is sharply demarcated from the darker medulla. The anterior and posterior lobes of the pituitary are also sharply demarcated from each other.

Nervous system

This part of the post-mortem examination may present difficulty for the less experienced prosector. The dog is placed on its sternum and a dorsal longitudinal mid-line skin incision made with a knife. The skin is reflected and the underlying muscles of the head and neck cut away with a knife.

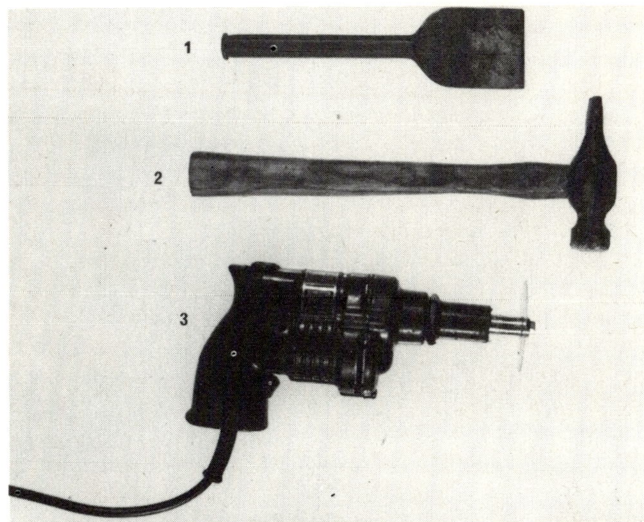

Fig. 4.7. Instruments for exposing the brain of dogs and cats. **1,** Steel chisel. **2,** Hammer.   **3,** Electrical oscillator necropsy saw. (Desoutter Bros Ltd, London.)

To examine the brain the calvaria must first be removed. For this an electrical oscillator saw may be used. An alternative method (the author's preference) in dogs is to use a steel chisel and hammer (*Fig.* 4.7). In either case approximately circular cuts are made around the exposed skull, beginning in the frontal sinuses and continuing round above the occipital condyles (*Fig.* 4.8). The calvaria is removed and the dura mater over the dorsal surface of the brain is incised with round-ended scissors. In cats

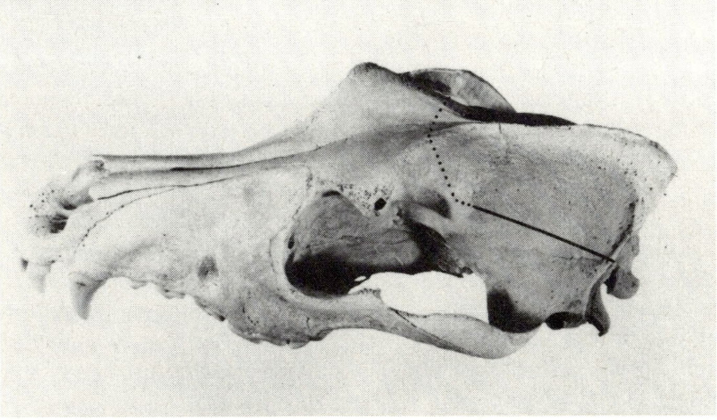

Fig. 4.8. Cranium of a dog showing the cuts required for removal of the calvaria to expose the brain.

it is necessary to remove the bony tentorium between cerebrum and cerebellum. The head is tipped forward on the nose and the brain stem is transected from the upper cervical spinal cord with a scalpel. The fingers or a scalpel handle are used to gently lift the ventral surface of the brain from the floor of the posterior fossa. Nerve roots are cut with scissors close to the cranial foramina and the brain can then be gently pulled from the anterior fossa with transection of the olfactory bulbs. Removal of the brain usually leaves the pituitary within its fossa: longitudinal scalpel incisions are made through the cavernous sinuses on both sides of the pituitary fossa. The gland can then be lifted out and fixed whole. The calvaria of puppies and kittens can be removed with strong scissors. The brain of these young animals is very soft so it is useful to fix the opened skull in situ for a few days before the brain is removed.

Removal of the spinal cord requires complete skinning of the dorsal surface of the body; the paravertebral muscles are then trimmed away with a knife and the ligamentum nuchae removed. Bone forceps are inserted into the canal of the first cervical vertebra and the lateral laminae cut. This is repeated along the length of the vertebral canal, holding the removed dorsal part of the column in the left hand while cutting with the right. At this stage it may be helpful to have the ventral surface of the spine supported, or flexed over the edge of the dissecting table. The lateral laminae should be removed as close as possible to the vertebral bodies, thus exposing the dorsal root ganglia and spinal nerves. An alternative approach to opening the spinal cord is to begin in the lumbosacral space and proceed in a cranial direction (Palmer, 1976). When the spinal cord is exposed the sacral dura mater is held with forceps and the cauda equina transected. The cord is held by forceps in the left hand and removed by cutting through the nerve roots so that they and the dorsal ganglia are included.

Tissue fixation

Naked eye examination of post-mortem tissues may have to be supplemented by histological examination. The important principles to remember for obtaining optimal preservation of tissues are as follows. Tissues should ideally be fixed as soon after death as possible. Autolytic changes occur rapidly in some organs (such as the pancreas and intestinal mucosa) and the rate of post-mortem change increases at higher temperatures. With tissues such as muscle, bone or skin post-mortem degeneration occurs more slowly so rapid fixation is less critical. Whenever possible bodies should be stored in a cool place prior to autopsy and, for many organs, useful necropsy information can be obtained up to 48 hours post mortem. This period will be shortened in warm weather and with obese animals in which subcutaneous fat provides insulation. Ideally corpses should be refrigerated at 4 °C. Deep freezing is not recommended: the slow freezing and thawing produces extensive artefactual changes that often render necropsy of little value.

Tissues for histological examination should be fixed in 10 per cent formal saline (*see* Appendix 2). The thickness of the blocks should not be more than 5–10 mm: formalin penetrates slowly and the interior parts of larger pieces of tissue fix poorly as a result. The volume of fixative should be greater than that of the specimen by a factor of five- or tenfold. Provided that thin blocks of tissue are fixed the area of tissue is limited only by the size of the microtome knife used for sectioning. Where focal lesions are present in an organ the sample selected for histological examination should also include normal tissue adjacent to the lesion. Where no naked-eye lesion is present the tissue sample should be a representative transverse section of the organ: tangential slices of organs such as the liver and kidney should be avoided. The site of tissue samples should be recorded for the pathologist and if more than one sample of an organ is submitted each should be labelled separately. This may be important if, say, more than one lymph node or different levels of the intestine are to be examined. Optimal fixation in formalin takes about a week provided that thin samples are taken. For small fragments of tissue, however, a few hours' fixation is adequate for subsequent processing to paraffin sections.

A practical consideration in fixing tissues for histology is always to use a wide-mouthed jar or bottle. Unfixed tissues are pliable and can be squeezed easily into a container with a narrow top such as a pill bottle. When the tissue is fixed, however, it is much less pliable and often cannot be withdrawn without first breaking the container.

Recording of post-mortem examinations

Ideally a concise description of the necropsy observations should always follow a post-mortem examination. This is particularly important in circumstances when litigation is a possibility. The descriptions should, briefly, be objective accounts of what was seen, palpated, measured or weighed. An attempt should be made to summarize the gross observations into a provisional macroscopic diagnosis (*see* Appendices 4, 5). It is often possible to do this without recourse to other investigations, although histological examination may be required for a definitive diagnosis. The principles underlying descriptions in pathology have been admirably summarized by Prichard (1966). These descriptions are of value not only to the clinician who may be asked to provide a formal report of his post-mortem examination but also to the histopathologist who may be asked to examine tissue specimens. Samples of pathology request and report forms are shown in Appendix 4. A suitable check-list of organ systems examined at necropsy is shown in Appendix 5.

REFERENCES

Palmer A. C. (1976) *Introduction to Animal Neurology,* 2nd ed. Oxford, Blackwell Scientific.
Prichard R. W. (1966) Descriptions in pathology. Avoiding pathological descriptions. *Path. Vet.* **3,** 169–77.

Chapter 5

Post-mortem and Agonal Changes

The small animal clinician carrying out a post-mortem examination is concerned to pick out those changes that are relevant to the animal's clinical history, or which may have contributed to its death. Recognition of these clinically pertinent changes of disease processes is often complicated by the presence of clinically irrelevant tissue changes. The ability to recognize the latter confidently is an important prerequisite for a sensible approach to necropsy work. Two types of artefactual changes may be seen in animal carcasses at necropsy — agonal and post-mortem changes.

AGONAL CHANGES

These take place in the short period immediately before death, that is just before or at the time of irreversible circulatory failure. The commonest change is vascular congestion: this is recognized most frequently in the lungs which may be darker and heavier than usual. Cutting into the lung allows blood to exude from the cut surfaces. Limited pulmonary oedema is a very common finding in the lungs of normal dogs and cats and is assumed to result from agonal impairment of venous return from the lungs to the atria. When death has occurred very suddenly, however, there may be only minimal congestion of the tissues.

A common agonal vascular change is seen in the pancreas in dogs: the gland is patchily or diffusely darkened with expansion of the interlobular connective tissue. The surface of the gland remains smooth and glistening and there are no gross signs of inflammation. Histological examination reveals only minimal interlobular oedema and extravasation of red blood cells, implying that the change occurred in the agonal period. Recognition of this common agonal change is important since it may be confused with pancreatic necrosis (synonyms: acute pancreatitis, necrotizing pancreatitis).

The latter is associated with other signs of necrosis and inflammation in the anterior abdomen, such as softening and calcification of the pancreas, peritoneal effusion with serosal hyperaemia and lipid droplet accumulation.

Agonal changes may also result from euthanasia, especially when barbiturates are used. Some of these changes are well recognized, others are less well appreciated. Barbiturate solutions are mildly irritant and produce hyperaemia at the sites of injection (around blood vessels, in the peritoneal, pericardial or pleural cavities). They also produce haemolytic darkening of the tissues around injection sites. When barbiturate solutions are injected into solid tissues a characteristic brown–red darkening may result (*Fig.* 5.1); similar changes may be seen on the pleura or peritoneum. Associated with this there may be the deposition of white crystalloid material resembling snow-flakes. This is most conspicuous in the heart after intracardiac euthanasia (*Fig.* 5.2).

The use of barbiturates for anaesthesia produces striking splenomegaly and this splenic distension is sometimes seen when these compounds are used for euthanasia. This is a variable feature, however, and it is not uncommon for there to be no alteration in spleen size in animals killed by the rapid intravenous injection of concentrated barbiturate solutions.

POST-MORTEM CHANGES

Post-mortem changes result from degradation of tissue components after the cessation of circulation. The changes are largely associated with autolytic degradation of cells by activation of their own lysosomal proteases and many of the resulting cellular and tissue alterations are similar to those that occur during ante-mortem tissue degeneration. This is an important point of practical concern in the histological examination of post-mortem tissues. For this reason it is important to know the interval of time that has elapsed between death of an animal and fixation of its tissues. Post-mortem changes may also result from multiplication of bacteria: organisms in the lumen of the bowel can proliferate not only in situ but will also pass into the body, frequently becoming widely distributed after death of the host animal. Factors which influence post-mortem changes include:

Rate of cooling of the carcass. Autolytic degradation of tissues results from enzymatic processes that are temperature-dependent. High body and ambient temperatures accelerate post-mortem degeneration.

Duration of post-mortem interval. Post-mortem changes can be detected microscopically in some organs within a few minutes of death. In many organs the degenerative changes are progressive with time and can become so advanced as to make post-mortem examination of very limited value.

Cause and mode of death. Generalized bacterial infection can be associated with rapid autolysis, especially if pyrexia has been present. Conversely, sudden death in a previously well animal may be followed by little complicating post-mortem change if reasonable care is taken.

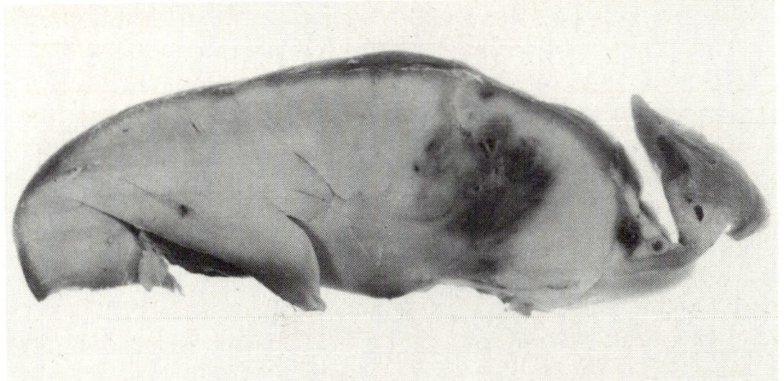

Fig. 5.1. Cut surface of the left ventricular myocardium of a puppy. The dark area in the upper part of the ventricle was produced by intramyocardial injection of barbiturate solution.

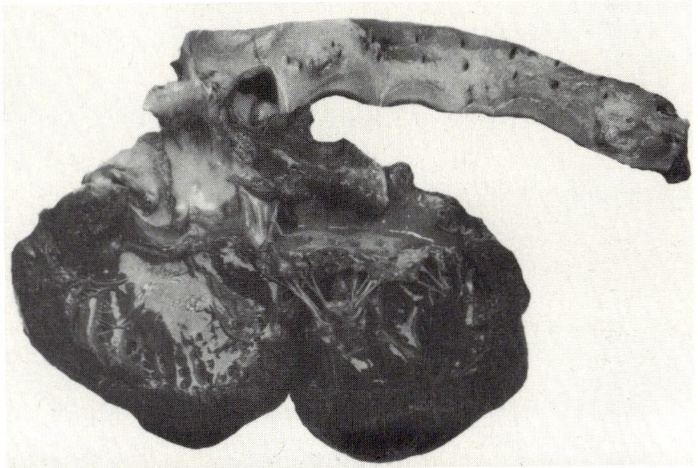

Fig. 5.2. White crystalloid appearance of ventricular endocardium in a dog killed by intracardiac injection of barbiturate solution.

The rate at which post-mortem changes occur varies with different tissues and the importance of this will vary with the kind of pathological investigation that may be required subsequently. Epithelia of the small intestine and kidney tubules, for example, undergo rapid post-mortem change: in the case of the former the change can be so rapid as to make almost worthless the examination of other than biopsy tissue in the histological investigation of malabsorption. Fortunately, with many tissues such as skin, bone and solid parenchymatous organs, the rate of post-mortem change is much lower so that necropsy can be usefully carried out up to 48 hours post mortem if reasonable care has been taken to cool the carcass. The practical implications of this can be summarized quite succinctly: dogs and cats should be examined as soon as possible after death. If necropsy is delayed the carcass should be stored in a refrigerator at temperatures of between 4 and 8 °C. *Carcasses should not be stored in the frozen state:* the process of freezing and thawing produces artefacts that usually render necropsy worthless. An additional objection is that thawing (at room temperature) of a frozen dog carcass can take up to several days. With large obese animals it can be useful to open the abdominal and thoracic cavities to accelerate cooling of the carcass: a moist cloth can be placed around the body to reduce drying of the exposed parts.

If critical histological examination of post-mortem tissues is contemplated it is useful to remove portions of the selected organs for fixation, even though the gross necropsy is to be carried out later. This can be extremely useful with samples of intestines, kidney and liver.

Post-mortem tissue alterations occur in three main categories:

    Changes in texture.
    Changes of colour.
    Tissue detachments.

Examples are summarized in Table 5.1 and discussed below.

Changes in texture

These result mainly from autolysis, but probably agonal alterations in hydration also play a part. The commonest change is a progressive autolytic softening of the tissues: this is most conspicuous in organs such as the kidney and liver. Post-mortem multiplication of bacteria in the bowel lumen and liver may be associated with gas formation, tympany, hepatic emphysema and the fetid smell of decomposition. In the eyes post-mortem changes lead to corneal opacity and scleral collapse so that the normal turgor of the globe is lost.

Changes of colour

These can be important causes of artefactual post-mortem appearance. The commonest example is the staining of tissues by haemoglobin that has leaked from red blood corpuscles into the extracellular environment. This produces an initial dulling of the surface and then a progressive reddening. This change is seen most conspicuously on the intima of large blood vessels, but a similar effect is seen on serosal and mucosal surfaces. Post-mortem haemoglobin staining accounts for the dull appearance of many organs in aborted fetuses. Haemoglobin staining of the small volumes of serosal fluid normally found in the pleural, pericardial and abdominal cavities may be mistaken for blood staining following ante-mortem haemorrhage.

Table 5.1. Summary of main post-mortem changes in small animals

	Texture	Colour	Detachments
Softening	Loss of characteristic firmness Softening, liquefaction (especially liver, kidney, brain, pancreas)	*Haemoglobin imbibition* Pink–red staining of intima of large blood vessels, serosae and serosal fluids *Bile staining* Yellow–green superficial discoloration of gallbladder, bile ducts, liver, intestines	Separation and sloughing of surface epithelium from small intestine, stomach (macroscopically visible) leads to thinning of wall of viscus with apparent increase in vascularity
Gas (a)	Intestinal and gastric tympany		
(b)	Gas bubbles Liver ('Aero chocolate') Blood vessels Beneath serosae	*Hypostatic congestion* Darkening and reddening of dependent parts – especially evident in lung and kidney; may also be seen on brain surface *Putrefaction* Green–black discoloration: especially in abdominal viscera and body wall	*Microscopic* detachments evident in glandular and ductular structures bronchi, urinary tract liver blood vessels (endothelium)

Darkening of tissues can also result from post-mortem pooling of blood — hypostatic congestion. This is usually a conspicuous feature of the lung, especially if the carcass has been lying on one side for more than a short period of time. The dependent lung is then usually heavier, firmer and darker than the lung that has been uppermost. Blood will exude from the cut surfaces of the dependent lung lobes. Similar but less impressive examples of hypostatic congestion may be recognized in other organs such as the kidneys.

Green–yellow discoloration of tissues adjacent to the biliary tract is a normal post-mortem change. Bile leaks through the lining of the tract and can produce discoloration of the adjacent surfaces of the liver and intestines.

Green–black discoloration of viscera and abdominal wall is a commonly recognized post-mortem change. This results from post-mortem growth of bacteria in the bowel lumen, and later in other organs. Hydrogen sulphide is formed by many bacteria: this reacts with iron in haemoglobin to form iron sulphide, giving rise to the characteristic discoloration of the decomposing carcass. The term 'pseudomelanosis' is sometimes used to describe the resulting colour change.

Tissue detachments

Tissue detachments or disaggregation lead to alterations in volume and texture of organs. They are recognized, at a gross level, most easily in the small intestine: detachment of mucosal epithelium from the underlying connective tissue of the lamina propria leads to loss of covering surface and thinning of the bowel wall. This change is progressive with time so that the bowel can eventually become thin-walled and transparent with a resulting increased prominence of intramural and subserosal blood vessels. This alteration is even more conspicuous in young animals and is accentuated if the viscera are distended by post-mortem gas formation. The resulting vascular prominence is frequently mistaken for evidence of enteritis. Detachment of intestinal mucosa can be recognized microscopically within a few minutes of cessation of circulation so that rapid fixation is absolutely essential for critical histological examination of intestinal samples.

Similar epithelial detachment occurs with other tissues and is easily recognized histologically, but rarely affects gross assessment of tissue changes since it is seldom as extensive or as advanced as in the small intestine. Structures that may be affected include gastric mucosa, ductal epithelium of the pancreatic and biliary tracts and mucosa of the large intestine. Detachment of epidermis is usually seen only when there is advanced post-mortem degeneration.

Chapter 6

Incidental Necropsy Findings

The previous chapter dealt with agonal and post-mortem alterations that may hinder the recognition of clinically relevant tissue changes. This chapter deals with non-artefactual appearances that are commonly found as incidental necropsy observations, and that generally appear to be of no clinical significance. Some of these appearances are due to normal physiological variations, some are anatomical features, others represent genuine lesions in the sense that they result from a pathological process. Changes of this last kind are often age-related in the sense that their prevalence is greater in older members of a species, breed or strain. In the older age group of a population the incidence of such 'background pathology' may reach relatively high levels and it is important that the small animal clinician be aware of this so that the clinical significance of a lesion can be given its proper weight. Since some of these senile changes occur in the abdominal cavity, can be appreciated on naked eye examination and by palpation, such an awareness is also of obvious concern to the surgeon.

Knowledge of 'background pathology' is of particular importance in species used in long term chronic toxicity studies and a great deal of information is available for the rat in which the incidences of many lesions are clearly related to age, sex and genetic strain of animal used (Burek, 1978). Quantitatively comparable data for non-rodent species are not available because of the greater genetic heterogeneity, but similar information is accumulating for the Beagle, since this breed of dog is commonly used in long term toxicity studies (Hottendorf and Hirth, 1974). Much of the information is about microscopic changes picked up in the systematic histological screening of tissues required for safety-testing purposes. These are not discussed further here: the scope of this chapter is generally restricted to those changes which can be recognized at a naked-eye level. They are considered according to the organ systems discussed in Chapter 4 on necropsy procedures.

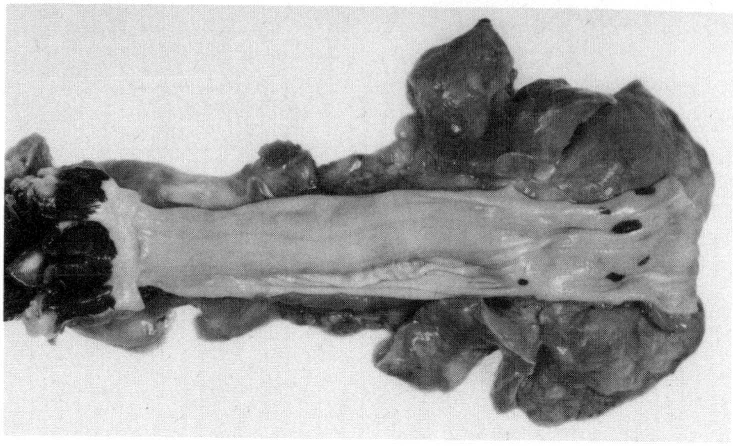

Fig. 6.1. Normal pigmentation of the pharynx and oesophagus in a Chow puppy.

ALIMENTARY SYSTEM

Mouth

Pigmentation of buccal mucosa is a feature that varies considerably between different breeds of dog. The Chow, for example, commonly has extensive dark buccal and pharyngeal pigmentation and this may extend into the oesophagus (*Fig.* 6.1). Nodular gingival hyperplasia (fibromatous epulis) is a common incidental finding in the older dog. This consists of smooth bulging gingival nodules close to the alveolar margins; cut surfaces are firm, white and fibrous with gritty foci.

Oesophagus

The epithelium of the normal oesophagus is corrugated longitudinally. In the lower third of the oesophagus in cats the epithelium forms distinct transverse folds. Occasionally in the dog the oesophageal epithelium bears multiple grey–black punctate elevations (*Fig.* 6.2). These result from distension of the ducts of the subepithelial mucus glands.

Peritoneum

Extensive omental and mesenteric haemorrhage can result from careless abdominal palpation. Older haemorrhage leads to tan discoloration of the omentum and peritoneum. Prolonged accumulation of blood (or other sterile fluids) within the abdominal cavity is also followed by a faint granular roughening of the serosal mesothelium.

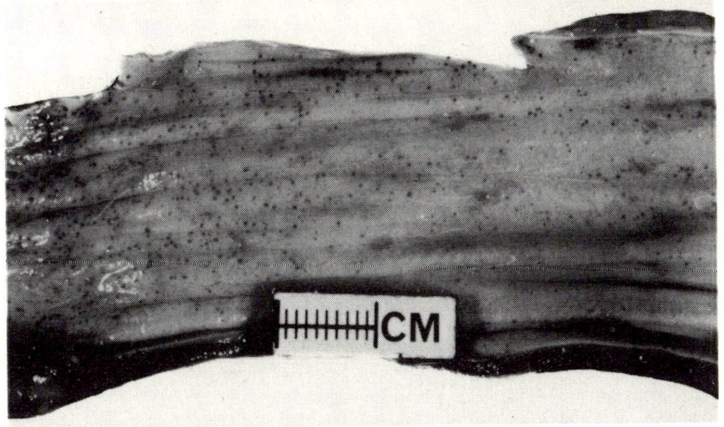

Fig. 6.2. Dark punctate foci caused by distended subepithelial mucus glands in the oesophagus of a dog.

Stomach

The normal stomach is lined by pale pink rugose mucous membrane. If food is present in the stomach the lining is darker, due to a physiological increase in mucosal blood flow: this should not be mistaken for gastritis. Stress ulcers are often found in the stomach of the dog and cat. These consist of multiple punctate flat haemorrhagic erosions or ulcers of the gastric mucosa and usually extend no more than a millimetre below the epithelial surface. Small amounts of blood may be visible on the mucosal surface. These lesions occur in association with a wide range of stressful situations and primary illnesses. They appear not to be of clinical significance *per se* in domestic animals although in some species they can lead to severe gastric haemorrhage.

Intramural fibroleiomyoma are not uncommon in the stomach of the aged dog: these are solitary, round submucosal fibrous nodules up to a few centimetres in diameter. They have firm cut surfaces, do not usually produce ulceration of the overlying mucosa and are of no clinical significance.

Intestines

The appearance of the intestines can vary under different physiological states: post-prandial hyperaemia occurs in the small intestine, as described for the stomach. Furthermore in the fasting state regional variation in the prominence of the mucosal blood vessels appears to be a normal feature. Linear darkening of the top of the intestinal mucosal folds is also a normal feature in dogs and cats. After the consumption of a fatty meal, such as

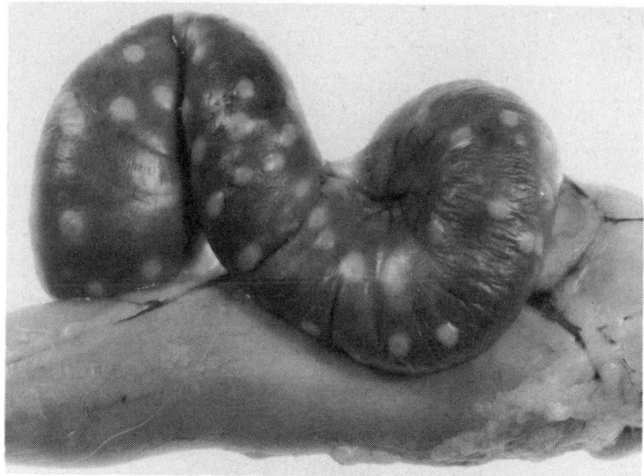

Fig. 6.3. Normal mucosal lymphoid tissue in the caecum of a 6-month-old Collie dog.

may be seen in puppies and kittens after suckling, the mesenteric lymphatic vessels become prominent as white cords that extend from the intestine to the local lymph nodes. Similar prominence of lymphatics may be seen in lean or cachectic dogs that have scanty deposits of mesenteric fat.

Lymphoid tissue can be very conspicuous in the alimentary tract of dogs and cats and may be found from the stomach to the anus. Miliary grey bulging nodules of mucosal and submucosal lymphoid tissue can be seen with the naked eye: they are often very conspicuous in the caecum, colon and rectum (*Fig.* 6.3) where they can be appreciated from the serosal aspect. Larger coalescing aggregations of lymphoid tissue occur in the upper small intestine where they are associated with flattening of the overlying mucosa. These may be up to several millimetres in diameter. These so-called 'pseudo-ulcers' can be appreciated radiographically in the live dog (O'Brien et al., 1969)

Liver

The liver of the older dog frequently contains one or more nodules of hyperplastic parenchyma (*Fig.* 6.4). These vary in size up to several centimetres in diameter, can be subcapsular or be situated in the deeper tissue, can be poorly demarcated from adjacent normal tissue, or can be sharply circumscribed. Frequently they are paler than normal liver tissue and may be mistaken for tumours. The pallor of the senile hyperplastic nodule is associated with the fat content of the constituent cells. These nodules are of no clinical significance. They do not seem to occur in the cat.

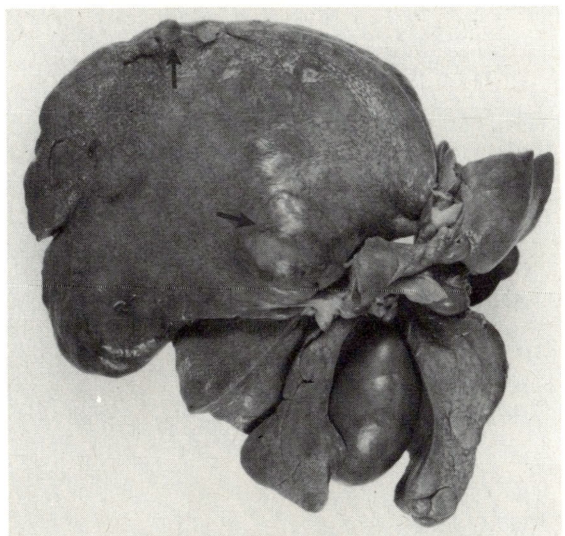

Fig. 6.4. Senile nodular hyperplasia in the liver of a 14-year-old Yorkshire Terrier. The nodules (arrows) vary in size and colour.

The normal biliary tract epithelium is smooth, glistening, green and flat. A common incidental senile change in the dog is cystic hyperplasia of the gallbladder mucosa: the epithelium is thrown into low fleshy folds that contain small cysts up to a few millimetres in diameter (*Fig.* 6.5). Small

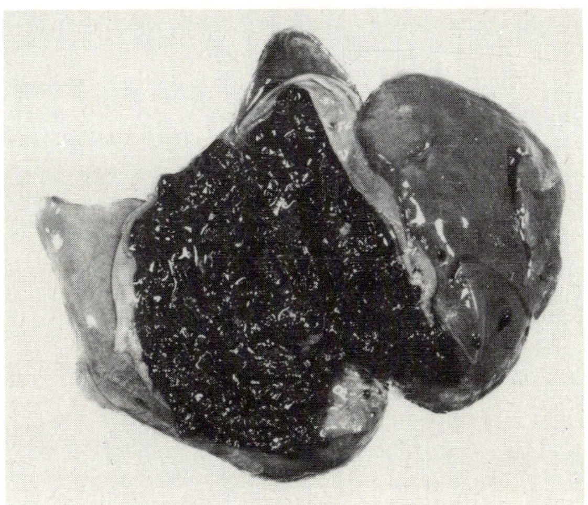

Fig. 6.5. Cystic hyperplasia of gallbladder mucosa (dog).

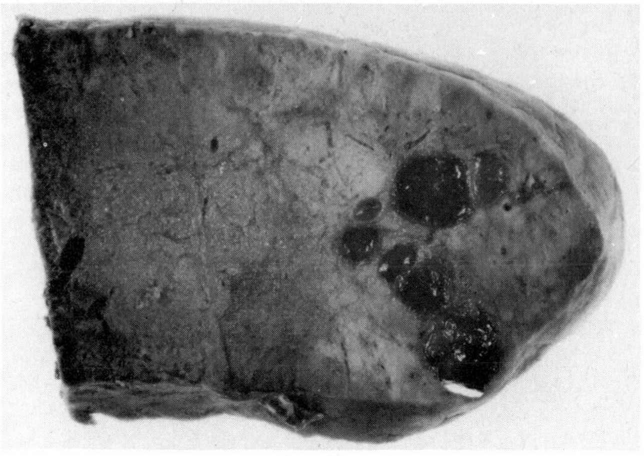

Fig. 6.6. Biliary cysts beneath the surface of the liver in a 14-year-old York-shire Terrier.

amounts of mucus are within the cysts and variable amounts of flocculent bile-stained mucus may be found in the bile. Small multiloculate biliary cysts are sometimes found in the liver. These vary in size up to a few millimetres in diameter, contain mucus or bile and are usually found in small clusters beneath the liver capsule. They are of no clinical importance (*Fig.* 6.6). The gallbladder may be distended in dogs that have not eaten recently.

Pancreas

In the pancreas senile nodular hyperplasia is a common incidental finding in both dog and cat. The normal pancreas has a uniform, well-defined lobular pattern. In the older animal there is often a variable nodularity of the external surface with compression of acinar tissue adjacent to the larger nodules that can be up to 1 cm in diameter.

In the cat it is not unusual to find interstitial pancreatitis: the gland has a finely granular surface and its cut surfaces are firmer and paler than usual. This appearance results from inflammation and fibrosis within the pancreas. It is not commonly associated with overt disease although clinical pancreatitis and hepatitis have been associated with this lesion (*Fig.* 6.7) (Kelly et al., 1975).

In the dog it is not uncommon to find foci of chalky white necrosis and calcification in the peripancreatic fat. This occurs in dogs with no history of pancreatitis: the cause is unknown and the lesion appears to be of no clinical significance. Punctate white foci are also often seen in the mesenteric, omental and perirenal adipose tissue of cats. The histological

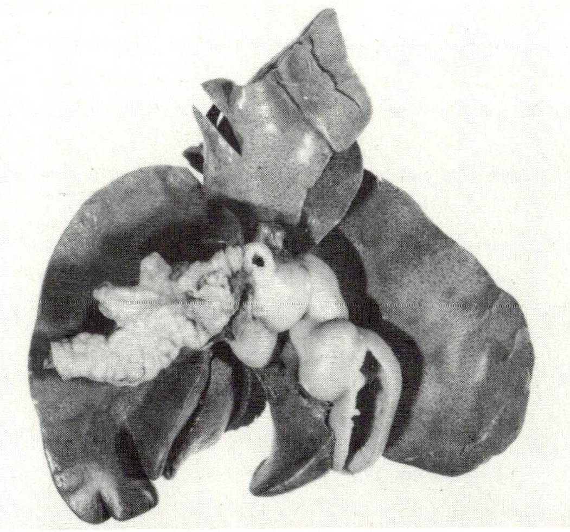

Fig. 6.7. Interstitial pancreatitis (cat). Note the fine granular appearance of the gland. (Reproduced by permission of the Editor of the *Journal of Small Animal Practice.*)

features of these foci are indistinguishable from those of pansteatitis, suggesting that subclinical forms of this condition are not infrequent.

UROGENITAL SYSTEMS

Kidney

Clinical renal disease is common in small animals so the practitioner and the pathologist are often required to examine the kidney. In the cat the renal capsule is always normally detached from the underlying cortex: if the capsule is cut the kidney immediately extrudes through the incision. This is not the case in dogs: it is common for there to be varying minor degrees of anatomical adhesion of the inner aspect of the capsule to the cortex. Removal of the capsule then tears parts of the superficial cortical tissue. This has to be distinguished from pathological adhesion of the capsule to the kidney when there is usually much firmer extensive or patchy adhesion. Focal radial scarring and atrophy is a relatively common incidental finding in the canine kidney: narrow wedges of pale shrunken cortex extend a variable distance from the capsular surface into the cortex and medulla. Histological examination of these radial scars shows glomerular and tubular atrophy, mild fibrosis and focal chronic inter-stitial inflammation. The changes are possibly a sequel to resolved mild focal pyelonephritis: there is rarely evidence to justify the description of infarction being applied to them. Solitary or multiple cysts can occasionally be found in the otherwise normal kidney of the cat and dog. These are probably of developmental origin and are of no functional significance.

A normal anatomical feature that should be emphasized for the small animal clinician is that the cortex of the feline kidney is much paler than that of the dog because it contains abundant intracytoplasmic lipid in the tubule cells of the nephron. The radial stellate vein pattern is normally conspicuous on the surface of the cat renal cortex. In both cat and dog there is often a conspicuous pale radial striated appearance of the medulla adjacent to the pelvis. This is a normal feature, but can be accentuated if there is any lesion such as tubular necrosis or if intratubular casts are present. Medullary calcification in the cat is common and may be recognized as white radial streaks.

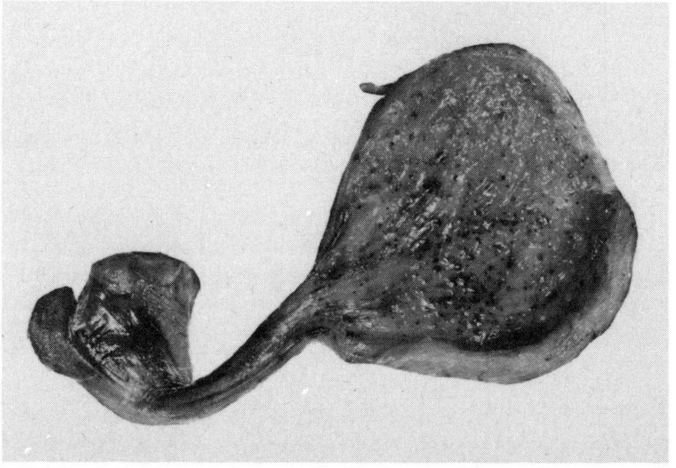

Fig. 6.8. Mild follicular cystitis (dog). The dark foci are reactive lymphoid follicles with surrounding hyperaemia.

Bladder

In the lower urinary tract of older dogs (especially in females) low grade cystitis is a relatively common incidental necropsy finding, sometimes associated with the presence of calculi. Cystitis is recognized by patchy roughening of the inner surface of the bladder. Subepithelial grey lymphoid follicles can also be seen elevating the bladder surface; they may be ringed by a narrow rim of hyperaemia (*Fig.* 6.8). Low grade cystitis may be present in the absence of clinical signs of urinary tract irritation or infection.

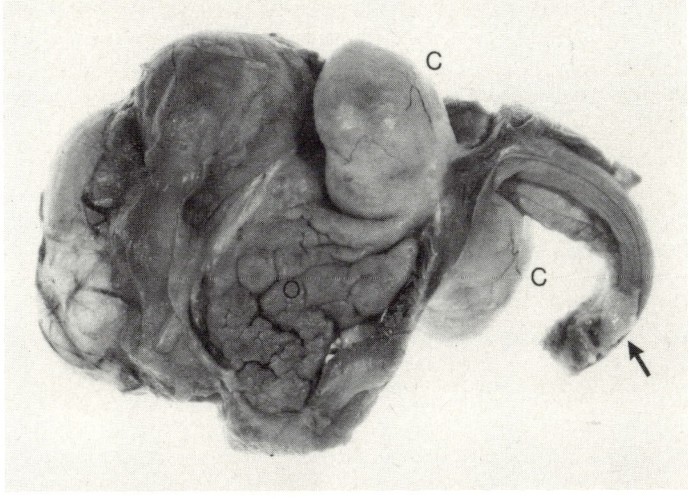

Fig. 6.9. Parovarian cysts (C) around the atrophic ovary (O) of an 8-year-old Labrador bitch. There is also a small mesometrial cyst (arrow).

Female genital tract

Ovary

Single or multiple parovarian cysts are very common in the older bitch. These can be up to 1 cm in diameter, are lined by smooth pale tissue and contain colourless fluid. The cysts can be situated on the surface of the ovary (*Fig.* 6.9) or be in the adjacent mesosalpinx or mesometrium. These common cysts are derived from mesothelium and are of no functional significance.

Uterus

Uterine changes may be related to normal cyclical activity or result from pregnancy. In the normal non-pregnant bitch there is post-oestral proliferation of the endometrium giving a fleshy and cystic appearance with a slight increase in the volume of uterine fluid (*Fig.* 6.10). After post-parturient involution the uterus remains loculated and the endometrium bears the dark pigmented transverse placental attachment sites. In the bitch small vaginal or uterine fibroleiomyoma may be found incidentally as pedunculated or intramural nodules up to a few millimetres in diameter (*Figs.* 6.11, 6.12). They are well circumscribed and fibrous and rarely cause clinical problems. The mesometrium may occasionally contain large lipomas.

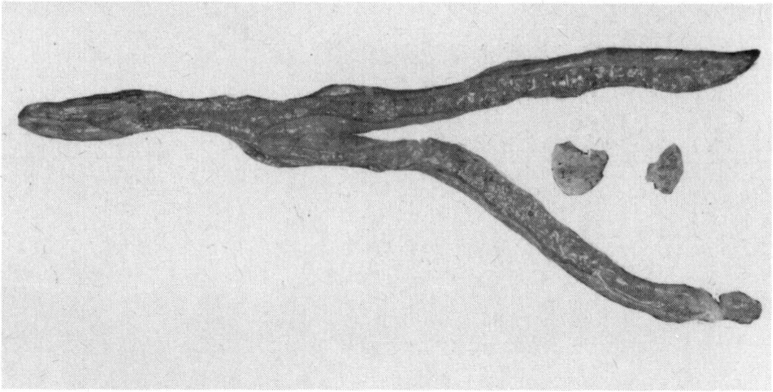

Fig. 6.10. Mild cystic endometrial proliferation in a post-oestral bitch.

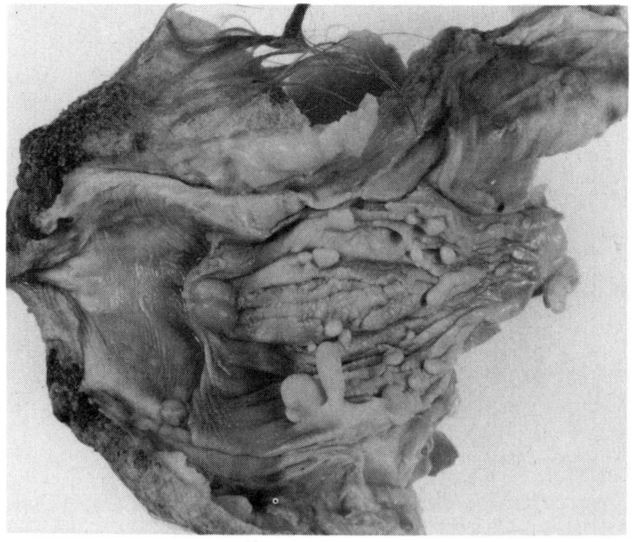

Fig. 6.11. Polypoid vaginal fibroleiomyomas in a 14-year-old Yorkshire Terrier bitch.

Mammary gland

Small mammary nodules are common incidental findings in the older bitch. These measure up to a few millimetres in diameter, are usually well circumscribed and hard. Localized areas of cystic dilatation of mammary ducts may also be found during random slicing of the mammary tissue.

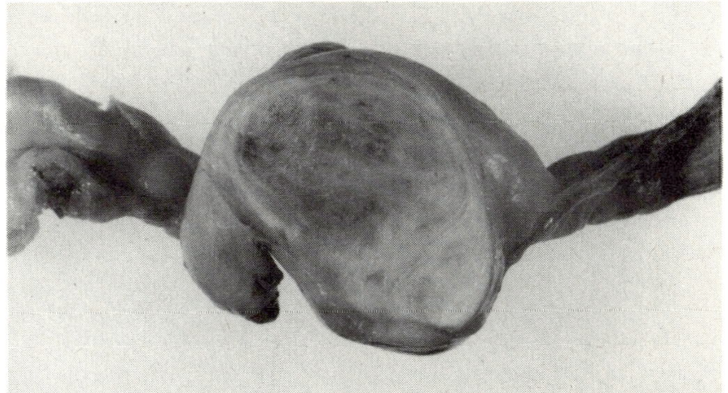

Fig. 6.12. A large uterine intramural fibroleiomyoma in an aged bitch (the same animal as illustrated in *Fig.* 6.11).

Male genital tract

Testes

The commonest incidental post-mortem finding in the dog is the presence of small testicular tumours. Interstitial cell nodules are the commonest: they are well circumscribed, reach a few millimetres in diameter and are tan–orange. Occasionally they have a darker red appearance because of telangiectatic change. Interstitial cell nodules may be classified as focal hyperplasia or as adenoma: the distinction is largely an arbitrary one without clinical importance since these lesions are entirely benign and without clinical effects, unless they enlarge sufficiently to distort the testes. Other testicular tumours (seminoma, Sertoli cell) are usually larger, paler and may produce distortion of the affected organ. Seminoma tend to be soft and homogeneous, Sertoli cell tumours may be firmer, but sometimes contain multiple small cysts. Retained testes in the inguinal canal or abdomen are more liable to develop Sertoli cell tumours and seminoma and to undergo torsion of the spermatic cord leading to infarction (Pearson and Kelly, 1975; Reif et al., 1979). Testicular lesions are rare in the cat.

Prostate

In the dog senile prostatic change is common. Irregular enlargement and nodular hyperplasia may produce palpable asymmetry. Cut surfaces of the enlarged prostate usually show irregular nodularity, but there is also frequently distension of the secretory structures to form multiloculate cysts. Enlargement of the prostate is frequently associated with nodular elevation of the adjacent urethral epithelium; this is usually evident when the urethra is opened from the bladder to the penis. Cut surfaces of the prostate of the mature dog sometimes have red, brown or yellow discoloration. This is associated with haemorrhage into the gland lumina and interstitium and the subsequent accumulation of haemosiderin and bilirubin. The pathogenesis of the extravasation is not known. In the castrated animal the prostate is considerably reduced in size.

Penis, prepuce

Examination of the penis and prepuce in the mature dog will usually reveal a small amount of turbid fluid in the preputial lumen. This low grade posthitis is often associated with hypertrophy of the preputial subepithelial lymphoid follicles which can be seen as multiple bulging miliary nodules.

RESPIRATORY TRACT

Upper airway

Focal grittiness is a very common finding in the cartilage of the larynx, trachea and bronchi of the old dog and cat. This is associated with both calcification and ossification; it can also be seen radiographically, but is of no clinical significance.

Narrowing of the trachea is a common anatomical feature in the toy breeds of dog. This is recognized as a reduction in the dorsoventral diameter of the trachea and flattening of the dorsal membrane. It is not usually of clinical significance unless very severe, or unless the dog is subjected to respiratory stress by exposure to high temperature and high humidity (O'Brien et al., 1966), or by palatine obstruction of the posterior pharynx.

Lungs

In the lungs the commonest incidental finding in dogs and cats is the presence of anthracosis due to inhalation of carboniferous materials from a polluted urban atmosphere. Anthracosis is easily recognized as black foci and striae beneath the pleura (*Fig.* 6.13), and around bronchi and larger pulmonary blood vessels. Drainage of the phagocytosed material can produce extensive blackening of bronchial lymph nodes. No clinically significant tissue reaction is provoked by the presence of this material in animal lungs. Localized areas of alveolar macrophage accumulation are common in cats. They are recognized as small pale subpleural foci. They consist microscopically of intra-alveolar foamy macrophages and probably result from reaction to inhaled lipid material.

In dogs and cats it is quite common to find limited areas of subpleural alveolar emphysema in the anterior lung lobes (*Fig.* 6.13). Quantitative

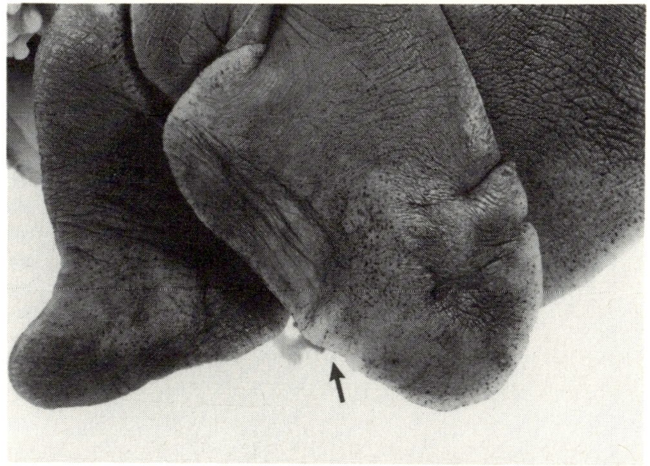

Fig. 6.13. Pleural anthracosis in the lung of a 14-year-old Yorkshire Terrier. The patchy pallor of the lung (arrow) results from localized alveolar emphysema.

assessment of this change has not been reported, but there is no clinical or pathological evidence to associate this limited destructive change with any deleterious effect on lung function. Palpation and slicing of the lungs of dogs will often reveal occasional subpleural punctate foci of intra-alveolar bone: the origin and significance of this ectopic bone is not known.

Dissection of the main stem bronchi in dogs and cats will often reveal a grossly visible increase in the amount of endobronchial secretion. This is usually clear and only slightly viscous. Interpretation of the significance of an apparent increase in bronchial secretions has to be assessed in the light of clinical evidence of bronchitis and histological evidence of goblet cell reaction. The amount of visible bronchial secretion in dogs and cats without clinical evidence of bronchitis seems to be extremely variable so the post-mortem diagnosis of bronchitis must be viewed with some critical reservation.

CARDIOVASCULAR SYSTEM

Heart

Nodular endocardiosis of the cardiac valves is the commonest incidental finding in the dog. The incidence of this change is clearly age-related (Jones and Zook, 1965) and some breeds, such as the Cocker Spaniel and Dachshund, appear to be particularly predisposed to the development of nodular endocardiosis (Buchanan, 1972). The lesion is recognized by variable degrees of thickening and opacification of the valve cusp with

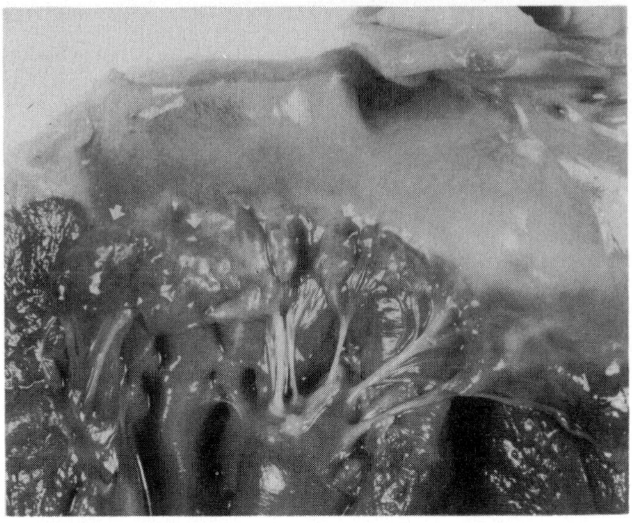

Fig. 6.14. Nodular endocardiosis of the mitral valve cusps (arrows). An incidental post-mortem finding in a 14-year-old mongrel dog.

nodularity of the cusp margin at the junction with the chordae tendineae (*Fig.* 6.14). The overlying endocardium is smooth without thrombotic roughening. The change is most commonly seen on the mitral valve, although the other cardiac valves can be affected. The tricuspid leaflets adjacent to the interventricular septum in the dog are normally slightly thicker and more opaque than the other cusps: this appearance can be mistaken for pathological change.

It should be emphasized that nodular endocardiosis is a very common incidental finding in dogs with no clinical evidence of cardiac dysfunction. Heart changes that may be associated with clinical cardiac dysfunction include myocardial hypertrophy, dilatation of the atrioventricular valve orifice, nodularity of the chordae tendineae, atrial dilatation, roughening or splitting of the left atrial endocardium (jet lesions) and focal scarring of the left ventricular papillary myocardium.

Focal or diffuse roughening of the atrial endocardium is occasionally seen as an incidental necropsy finding in dogs (*Fig.* 6.15). It is associated with splitting and calcification of endocardial elastic fibres: the underlying pathogenesis and possible clinical significance are unknown.

Blood vessels

Clinically significant primary disease of large blood vessels is uncommon in dogs and cats but focal lesions of arterial intima are common incidental

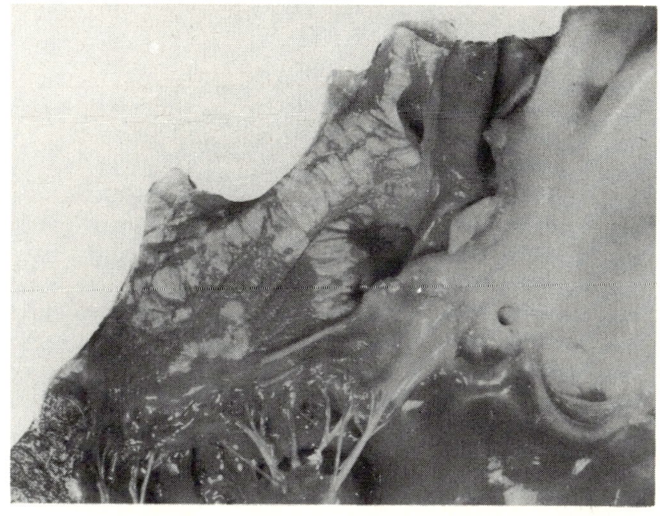

Fig. 6.15. Patchy calcification of left atrial endocardium (dog).

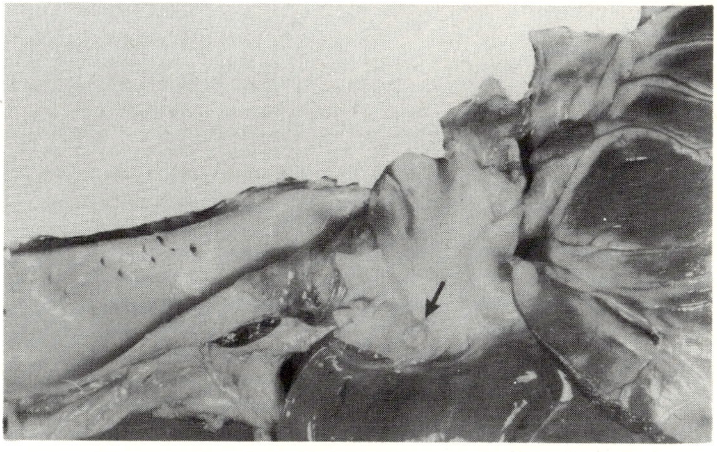

Fig. 6.16. A plaque of calcified aortic intima (arrow) (dog).

necropsy findings. These are recognized as punctate elevations of the intima of the aortic (*Fig.* 6.16) or pulmonary arterial trunks; the overlying surface is smooth and without thrombotic roughening. Beneath the intima is gritty white material: this often consists of calcified debris, but ectopic cartilage and bone are also found at these sites.

LYMPHORETICULAR SYSTEM

Spleen

Two senile changes occur in the spleen of the dog so frequently that they may confuse the small animal clinician, especially when discovered at laparotomy.

Siderofibrosis of the splenic capsule and trabecular connective tissue is seen in a large proportion of dogs older than 2 years (Ishmael and Howell, 1967). This is recognized as plaques of opaque roughened pale or yellow tissue on the external surfaces, edges and cut surfaces of the organ. The change results from accumulation of haemosiderin and haematoidin, together with variable fibrosis. The change is of no clinical importance.

Lymphoid hyperplasia of the canine spleen is recognized by the presence of one or more bulging subcapsular nodules that can be up to several centimetres in diameter. The nodules consist of soft grey–red tissue that blends into the adjacent splenic pulp. The pathogenesis of this common senile change is unknown: there is no evidence to associate this form of nodular lymphoid hyperplasia with either infection or leukaemia. Although lymphoid hyperplasia can produce striking asymmetrical enlargement of the spleen the change appears to have no deleterious clinical effect. Both siderofibrosis and nodular hyperplasia can coexist in the same organ: neither change constitutes an indication for splenectomy.

Ectopic splenic nodules occur occasionally in the omentum or on the surface of the spleen. They are usually small (less than 2 mm in diameter), round nodules of dark tissue resembling splenic pulp. In the dog the spleen sometimes has a deeply fissured appearance of the capsule with fibrous thickening of the adjacent tissue. The origin of this is unclear: the possibility of earlier trauma does not usually have historical support.

Lymph nodes

Age-related change in the size of lymphoid tissue is striking in the dog and cat. The gradual involution of the thymus is a well-recognized age-related phenomenon but comparable changes in lymph nodes and tonsil are not so clearly appreciated. In general, lymph nodes are relatively larger in the young animal and follicular tissue is more conspicuous in the tonsils and splenic white pulp, the latter sometimes giving a distinct miliary appearance to the cut surfaces of these organs. With increasing age the lymphoid tissue becomes less prominent. Failure to recognize this age-related change often results in lymph nodes of puppies and kittens being clinically assessed as enlarged, when they are well within the normal range for the age.

Abnormal coloration of lymph nodes can result from haemosiderosis, melanosis, anthracosis and accumulation of tattoo ink pigment. The nodes are discoloured but not enlarged. Tan–brown discoloration of nodes occurs in any region where there is extravasation of blood; the underlying cause of the haemorrhage is usually not difficult to assess. In the dog the lymph node situated near the pancreatic flexure commonly has a distinct tan appearance because haemosiderin accumulates within macrophages in the node. The cause of this very common pigmentation is not clear. Melanotic grey or black discoloration of lymph nodes can be seen adjacent to chronic skin lesions, particularly if there is pruritus and prolonged scratching. Persistent self-induced trauma to the pigmented skin surface leads to liberation of epidermal melanin: this is phagocytosed by macrophages that then accumulate in the drainage lymph nodes as part of the changes of dermatopathic lymphadenopathy. Similar lymph node changes can occur in the vicinity of heavily pigmented melanotic tumours: the melanin is released from the tumour cells and drains to the local lymph node. Thus, darkening of a node is not an invariable sign of metastatic spread from a putative melanoma.

Blackening of bronchial lymph nodes by anthracotic pigment is an extremely common finding in the thorax of urban animals. A similar darkening of lymph nodes occurs where skin tattooing has been carried out for identification purposes. Because the amount of pigment is small the change is not always grossly apparent in the drainage lymph node, although it can be appreciated easily on histological examination.

ENDOCRINE SYSTEM

Adrenals

The adrenal glands should be dissected out intact with their retroperitoneal fat and fixed whole at least overnight so that hardening occurs. The fat surrounding the glands can then be removed and the partially fixed adrenals sliced carefully with a scalpel. Cutting of unfixed adrenals, especially if a sharp knife is not used, usually results in crushing and distortion of the tissue. The method suggested is also to be preferred since few clinical conditions of the adrenals can be diagnosed with any confidence solely on the gross appearance of the glands.

In the cat calcification of the cortex is extremely common, producing pale gritty foci easily appreciated on cutting. There is no evidence to suggest that this change is of any functional significance and it is not associated with soft tissue calcification in other sites.

In the older dog there is commonly nodular hyperplasia of the adrenal cortex. Nodules of pale cortical tissue (up to a few millimetres diameter) bulge through the capsule giving the external surface of the gland a botryoid (grape-like) appearance. Cutting of the glands usually reveals that this nodular tissue also extends into the adrenal medulla. The change is always bilateral. The size of the glands may be increased. This common senile change is usually non-functional: a retrospective diagnosis of Cushing's disease cannot be made on the basis of finding enlarged nodular adrenal

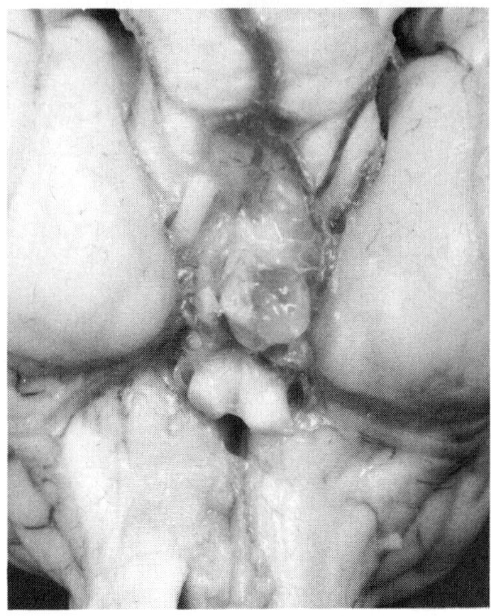

Fig. 6.17. Small congenital cyst on the ventral aspect of the anterior pituitary (dog).

glands, neither are the histological features of the hyperplastic glands sufficiently distinctive to justify an inference about the functional state of the tissue (Kelly et al., 1971).

Tumours of the adrenal medulla (phaeochromocytoma) are occasional incidental findings in old dogs. They cause unilateral enlargement of the gland and the medulla is expanded by soft tissue that has a characteristic dark tan appearance. Fixation of phaeochromocytoma produces brown darkening of the fixing fluid. These tumours generally appear to be non-functional.

Thyroids

Small nodules and cysts are found in the elderly cat. These incidental findings are of no clinical significance (Lucke, 1964).

Pituitary

Small developmental cysts (up to a few millimetres in diameter) are common in the pituitary of the dog. They can be seen on the surface of the gland after the brain is removed. They have transparent fluctuating walls and contain clear colourless fluid (*Fig.* 6.17). They are usually of no clinical significance, although large cysts of this kind have been described in Alsatians with pituitary dwarfism (Allan et al., 1978).

NERVOUS SYSTEM

The dura mater of the brain and spinal cord is normally opaque and grey. The spinal cord can be removed from the vertebral canal with the dura mater intact, but the brain cannot be removed without first incising and reflecting the overlying dura. Plaques of bone and marrow are commonly found in the spinal dura mater of dogs, particularly in the larger breeds. These plaques are usually lanceolate, measure up to a few millimetres in length and can be distributed throughout the length of the cord. Their colour varies from grey to pink, depending on the amount of marrow that is present. Flat plaques of dural bone usually produce no harmful effects but nodular accumulations can compress spinal cord and nerve roots. This condition is also called ossifying pachymeningitis, but there is no evidence to support the idea that the lesion is of inflammatory origin.

The leptomeninges of the cerebral hemispheres are often thickened and opaque in the older dog. This is most obvious in the sulci of the dorsal surface of the hemispheres, adjacent to the median fissure. The appearance results from mild leptomeningeal fibrous thickening and is not to be confused with meningitis: the latter is relatively uncommon in carnivores, is associated with other signs of meningeal inflammation (exudation, hyperaemia) and tends to be most obvious on the ventral surface of the brain.

SKELETAL SYSTEM

Osteoarthritis (syn. osteoarthrosis, 'arthritis', degenerative joint disease) is a common incidental finding in the older dog, in the absence of clinical evidence of locomotor abnormality. This finding is more common in the larger breeds and is most commonly recognized in the large joints, such as the shoulder, stifle and hip. Osteoarthritis is represented by a range of articular and periarticular changes that can affect both hard and soft tissues. The joint capsule may be thickened by fibrous connective tissue. This is recognized most often in the hip. Articular cartilage may be fibrillated, eroded or eburnated. Periarticular osteophyte proliferation may be present, or there may be cartilaginous proliferation at the zone of transitional synovium adjacent to the articular cartilage. This last change is seen most commonly adjacent to the femoral condyles and on the acetabular rim. In the toy breeds flattening of the femoral condyles is a common feature and this may also be associated with cartilaginous metaplasia of the adjacent synovium. Assessment of the possible clinical significance of degenerative joint disease in dogs is subjective: a large proportion of dogs, especially in the larger breeds, are found to have osteoarthritic lesions at necropsy — in the absence of any clinical evidence of joint disease. This is in contrast to the situation in the cat, in which lesions of osteoarthritis are uncommon.

REFERENCES

Allan G. S., Huxtable C. R. R., Howlett C. R. et al. (1978) Pituitary dwarfism in German Shepherd dogs. *J. Small Anim. Pract.* **19,** 711–27.

Buchanan J. W. (1972) Spontaneous left atrial rupture in dogs. *Adv. Exp. Med. Biol.* **22,** 315–34.

Burek J. D. (1978) *Pathology of Ageing Rats.* Boca Raton, CRC Press.

Hottendorf G. H. and Hirth R. S. (1974) Lesions of spontaneous subclinical disease in Beagle dogs. *Vet. Path.* **11,** 240–58.

Ishmael J. and Howell J. Mc C. (1967) Siderofibrotic nodules of the spleen in the dog. *J. Small Anim. Pract.* **8,** 501–10.

Jones T. C. and Zook B. C. (1965) Ageing changes in the vascular system of animals. *Ann. NY Acad. Sci.* **127,** 671–84.

Kelly D. F., Gaskell C. J. and Baggott D. G. (1975) Jaundice in the cat associated with inflammation of the biliary tract and pancreas. *J. Small. Anim. Pract.* **16,** 163–72.

Kelly D. F., Siegel E. T. and Berg P. (1971) The adrenal gland in hyperadrenalo-corticism. A pathologic study. *Vet. Path.* **8,** 385-400.

Lucke V. M. (1964) An histological study of thyroid abnormalities in the domestic cat. *J. Small Anim. Pract.* **5,** 351–8.

O'Brien J. A., Buchanan J. W. and Kelly D. F. (1966) Tracheal collapse in the dog. *J. Am. Vet. Radiol. Assoc.* **7,** 12–20.

O'Brien T. R., Morgan J. P. and Lebel J. L. (1969) Pseudoulcers in the duodenum of the dog. *J. Am. Vet. Med Assoc.* **155,** 713–16.

Pearson H. and Kelly D. F. (1975) Testicular torsion in the dog: a review of 13 cases. *Vet. Rec.* **97,** 200–4.

Reif J. S., Maguire T. S., Kenney R. M. et al. (1979) A cohort study of canine testicular neoplasia. *J. Am. Vet. Med. Assoc.* **175,** 719–23.

Appendix 1

Clinical Pathology and Haematology

Appendix 1.1. Chymotrypsin Assay for the Estimation of Exocrine Pancreatic Function (PABA–Peptide Test)

The test is based on the rapid hydrolysis of a synthetic peptide, benzoyl-tyrosyl-p-aminobenzoic acid (BT-PABA) by pancreatic chymotrypsin with the release of p-aminobenzoic acid (PABA). Following oral administration of BT-PABA, an estimation of chymotrypsin activity can be made by measuring subsequent PABA levels in blood or urine.

A solution is made up containing 3·5 mmol (1·65 g) per litre of BT-PABA (Fluorochem Ltd, Glossop, Derbyshire).

Procedure

1. Withhold food from dog overnight.
2. Take 2 ml sample of blood into EDTA or fluoride tube (time 0).
3. Administer BT-PABA solution through a stomach tube at a dose of 10 ml/kg body weight.
4. Take further 2 ml samples of blood (EDTA or fluoride) at 1 and 2 hours following dosing (alternatively PABA levels may be measured in urine produced over the first 6 hours following dosing).

Note: this test can be combined with the xylose absorption test (Appendix 1.2).

REFERENCE

Batt R. M., Bush B. M. and Peters T. J. (1979) A new test for the diagnosis of exocrine pancreatic insufficiency in the dog. *J. Small Anim. Pract.* **20**, 185–92.

Appendix 1.2. Xylose Absorption Test

The test is based on the absorption of a sugar, D(+) xylose, by the small intestine and the subsequent measurement of xylose levels in the blood.

A 5 per cent solution of xylose is used.

Procedure

1. Withhold food from the dog overnight.
2. Take 2 ml sample of blood into a fluoride tube (time 0).
3. Administer xylose solution through a stomach tube (or mixed with a very small quantity of meat) at a dose of 0·5 g (10 ml)/kg body weight.
4. Take further 2 ml samples of blood (fluoride) at 30, 60, 90 and 120 min following dosing.

Note: this test can be combined with the PABA Test (Appendix 1.1).

REFERENCE

Hill F. W. G., Kidder D. E. and Frew J. (1970) A xylose absorption test for the dog. *Vet. Rec.* **87**, 250–5.

Appendix 1.3. Intestinal Biopsy

While the use of a peroral biopsy capsule has been described in the dog, samples are usually taken at laparotomy. The gross appearance of the bowel may be normal even in the presence of severe malabsorption. Lesions may not be evenly distributed and thus at least three full-thickness, longitudinally elliptical biopsies (duodenum, jejunum and ileum) should be taken. Care should be taken to avoid Peyer's patches, as histological interpretation of these areas may be difficult. Samples should be submitted in formol saline for histological examination. Sophisticated techniques for assessing mucosal enzyme levels have been described but are not routinely available.

Appendix 1.4. Water Restriction Test

This test assesses the ability of the kidneys to concentrate urine following a period of water deprivation. It should never be carried out in the presence of uraemia, nor continued for longer than 8 hours without close supervision.

Procedure

1. Food and water are withdrawn, the animal is weighed and the bladder emptied.

2. The animal is re-weighed after 8 hours and the bladder emptied again.

3. A further urine sample is taken a short while later. If the urine specific gravity has risen to > 1020 the kidneys are capable of concentrating urine and the test can be stopped; if there has been no concentration of urine and the animal has lost 3–5 per cent of body weight, the kidneys are not capable of concentration and the test should be terminated. If there has been little concentration of urine or loss in bodyweight and the animal is well, sampling and weighing should be repeated after a further 4 hours.

Appendix 1.5. Paracentesis

A small area of the ventral abdominal wall just behind the umbilicus is prepared surgically. A 21 gauge needle is introduced through the skin in the midline, moved 1 cm caudally and passed through the linea alba into the peritoneal cavity. If a larger gauge needle, or needle and catheter (e.g. Plextrocan, Portex Ltd, Kent) is used, the skin and abdominal wall should be infiltrated with local anaesthetic. The procedure can be carried out with the animal standing or restrained in lateral recumbency.

Appendix 1.6. Bromsulphthalein (BSP) Retention Test

The test measures the ability of the liver to remove a dye, bromsulphthalein (BSP), from the circulation following intravenous injection.

Procedure

1. A 10 ml blood sample (control) is taken into a heparin tube.

2. BSP (Hynson, Westacott & Dunning Inc., Baltimore, Maryland, USA) is injected intravenously as a 5 per cent solution at a dose of 5 mg/kg bodyweight, taking care that all the solution goes into the vein.

3. A further 10 ml blood sample (heparin) is taken 30 minutes later from a different vein.

Note: care must be taken not to contaminate the initial control blood sample with BSP; the solution for injection should preferably be prepared by someone other than the person taking the sample.

Appendix 1.7. Thoracentesis

Thoracentesis is best carried out with the animal standing or in sternal recumbency, using gentle manual restraint and local anaesthesia. Mild tranquillization or sedation may be necessary but animals with considerable amounts of pleural fluid will not tolerate general anaesthesia. Clinical and radiographic information will usually dictate which side of the pleural cavity to tap; if both sides are equally involved, the right side is usually preferable. An area of skin is prepared surgically over the 6th, 7th and 8th intercostal (i.c.) spaces approximately one-third of the way up the chest wall. Local anaesthetic is infiltrated into the skin approximately 2 cm caudal to the 7th i.c. space and in the subcutaneous tissues forward to this i.c. space where the intercostal muscles and pleura are also in-filtrated. A 19 G or 20 G needle, attached via a three-way stopcock to a syringe, is introduced through the skin, directed forward and then medially through the anaesthetized intercostal muscles and parietal pleura. To avoid the intercostal vessels, the needle should be passed through the caudal part of the intercostal space, but this is difficult to judge in small dogs and cats. Where the fluid is viscous, e.g. some cases of exudative pleurisy, or where the chest is to be drained by thoracentesis, a larger gauge catheter is preferable, usually introduced over the needle, e.g. Plextrocan (Portex Ltd, Hythe, Kent). Where such a catheter is used, a small incision should be made in the anaesthetized skin before intro-duction to avoid 'rucking up' the leading edge of the catheter.

Appendix 1.8. Pericardiocentesis

The methods of restraint, preparation of the skin and introduction of local anaesthetic are similar to those used for thoracentesis (Appendix 1.7.). The left side of the chest is invariably used and the site of intro-duction of the catheter or needle is usually the sixth intercostal space in the lower third of the chest wall.

A catheter, introduced over a needle, e.g. Plextrocan (Portex Ltd, Kent) is preferable as it is both longer than an ordinary hypodermic needle and blunt-ended, and the need is usually for drainage as well as sampling. Alternatively a longer, but usually narrower gauge, catheter may be introduced into the pericardium through a needle, giving even less risk of displacement during drainage.

Following local anaesthesia the needle is introduced through a small skin incision, directed forward to the 6th intercostal space and passed medially through the chest wall, across the pleural space (which is minimal in gross pericardial effusion) and through the pericardium. When fluid returns along the needle, the catheter should be advanced into the peri-cardium and the needle withdrawn.

Appendix 1.9. Bone-marrow Biopsy

In the dog bone-marrow samples are most easily obtained from the iliac crest under local anaesthesia with or without sedation. An area over the iliac crest is prepared surgically and infiltrated with local anaesthetic. A small skin incision is made and a 16 G or 18 G bone-marrow biopsy needle (e.g. Rosenthal Needle, Becton Dickinson UK Ltd, Wembley, Middx) introduced by steady pressure and rotation into the anterior–dorsal aspect of the iliac crest. The stylet is removed and suction applied with a 20 ml syringe. The suction is stopped as soon as marrow appears in the syringe to avoid dilution of the sample with blood. Smears of marrow are made as clean, dry glass slides and quickly dried by waving them in the air.

In the cat, while the iliac crest may be used, marrow may be more easily obtained from the femur. The cat is anaesthetized, an area over the trochanteric fossa prepared surgically, and a small skin incision made. The leg is held firmly in one hand and an 18 G biopsy needle introduced into the medulla of the femur through the trochanteric fossa. Marrow is aspirated and smears made as above. Intravenous needles (18 G) may be used to obtain biopsies but, in the absence of stylets, tend to become plugged with bone.

Failure to obtain a satisfactory sample of marrow may be due to incorrect placement of the needle but may in some cases be due to a real absence of active marrow. Interpretation of bone-marrow smears requires some experience.

Appendix 1.10. Bleeding Time

A small incision is made, using either a standard lancet stab or a scalpel blade, in the pinna of the ear. The inner or outer surface may be used but it must be shaved and clean. Blood is removed gently every 15 seconds using, for example, the edge of a filter paper, and the time noted when bleeding ceases. Care must be taken in removing blood that the forming platelet plug is not dislodged.

Appendix 1.11 Glucose Tolerance Test

This test, which relies on normal intestinal absorption, measures the degree and persistence of the rise in plasma glucose levels following oral administration of glucose.

A 12.5 per cent solution of glucose is used.

Procedure

1. Withhold food from the dog overnight.
2. Take 2 ml sample of blood into fluoride tube (time 0).
3. Administer glucose solution through a stomach tube (or mixed with a very small quantity of meat) at a dose of 2 g (16 ml)/kg bodyweight.
4. Take further 2 ml samples of blood (fluoride) at 30, 60, 90 and 120 minutes following dosing.

REFERENCE

Hill F. W. G. and Kidder D. E. (1972) The oral glucose tolerance test in canine pancreatic malabsorption. *Br. Vet. J.* **128**, 207–14.

Appendix 1.12. Reference (Normal) Values

Haematology

	Dog		Cat	
Packed cell volume (PCV) (%)	40–50		30–35	
Red blood cell (RBC) count ($10^6/\mu$l)	5·1–6·8		5·5–7·5	
Haemoglobin concentration (g/100 ml)	12·0–16·5		9·8–12·7	
Mean corpuscular volume (MCV) (fl)	65–75		40–55	
Mean corpuscular haemoglobin concentration (MCHC) (%)	31–35		30–35	
Total white blood cell (WBC) count ($10^3/\mu$l)	8·5–14·0		10·0–22·0	
	Abs.	Diff.	Abs.	Diff.
Band (young) neutrophils	—	< 3	0·1 ± 0·2	1
Neutrophils (mature)	8·3 ± 0·8	74	8·7 ± 4·5	60
Lymphocytes	2·3 ± 0·6	20	3·7 ± 2·1	28

	Dog		*Cat*	
	Abs.	Diff.	Abs.	Diff.
Eosinophils	0·2 ± 0·2	2	1·2 ± 1·0	9
Monocytes	0·5 ± 0·3	4	0·2 ± 0·2	2
Basophils	Uncommon	0	Uncommon	0
Platelet count ($10^5/\mu$l)	2–9		3–7	

Notes
   1. Abs. = absolute ($10^3/\mu$l); Diff. = differential (%).
   2. These values should be used as guidelines only; considerable variations occur in some parameters, e.g. WBC count, in normal animals.
   3. PCV will be artifically lowered by under-filling the sample tube.
   4. PCV is higher in Greyhound-type dogs (c. 55 per cent).
   5. Young animals ($<$10 months) frequently show a lymphocytosis and may have lower PCV and haemoglobin values.

Blood biochemistry

	Dog	*Cat*
Urea (mmol/l)	2·5–6·7	5·0–10·0
Urea nitrogen (mg/dl)	7–20	15–30
Creatinine (μmol/l)	80–175	80–175
Glucose (mmol/l)	3·0–5·0*	3·3–5·0*
Total protein (g/l)	62–75	60–75
Albumin (g/l)	30–40	30–40
Bilirubin (μmol/l)	0–5	0–4
Cholesterol (mmol/l)	3·1–6·5	1·8–3·9
Ammonia (μmol/l)	$<$50	–
Alkaline phosphatase (SAP) (i.u.)	21–106	20–110
Glutamate pyruvate transaminase (SGPT) (i.u./l)	10–20	10–20
Creatine phosphokinase (CPK) (i.u./l)	$<$40	$<$40
Amylase (i.u./l)	800–2000	800–2000
Sodium (mmol/l)	135–150	115–150
Potassium (mmol/l)	3·5–4·5	2·5–3·9
Chloride (mmol/l)	102–112	117–123
Calcium (mmol/l)	2·4–2·9	1·8–2·5
Inorganic phosphorus (mmol/l)	0·6–1·1	1·2–2·0

Note
This table of 'normal' values is intended for reference only. Differences in analytical methods may produce significant differences in 'normal', or reference, ranges and the clinician should obtain such reference values from the laboratory concerned. Similarly, no indication has been given of changes due to age or sex, though where this is likely to be marked, reference has been made to this in the text.

   *Values quoted are for plasma glucose; measurements made using whole blood are some 12 per cent lower.

Appendix 1.13. Blood Biochemistry — Conversion Factors

The international system of units (SI) has been adopted as the most consistent means of expressing biochemical, and other, values. The following are the conversion factors from previously used units for the measurements referred to in this book.

Urea	mmol/l $\times$ 6·02 = mg/100 ml mg/100 ml $\times$ 0·166 = mmol/l blood urea nitrogen (BUN) (mg/100 ml) $\times$ 2·14 = blood urea (mg/100 ml)
Glucose	mmol/l $\times$ 18 = mg/100 ml mg/100 ml $\times$ 0·056 = mmol/l
Xylose	mmol/l $\times$ 15 = mg/100 ml mg/100 ml $\times$ 0·067 = mmol/l
Creatinine	μmol/l $\times$ 0·0113 = mg/100 ml mg/100 ml $\times$ 88·4 = μmol/l
Protein	g/l $\times$ 0·1 = g/100 ml g/100 ml $\times$ 10 = g/l
Bilirubin	μmol/l $\times$ 0·0585 = mg/100 ml mg/100 ml $\times$ 17·1 = μmol/l
Cholesterol	mmol/l $\times$ 38·7 = mg/100 ml mg/100 ml $\times$ 0·026 = mmol/l
Ammonia	μmol/l $\times$ 1·7 = μg/100 ml μg/100 ml $\times$ 0·588 = μmol/l
Alkaline phosphatase (SAP)	i.u./1 $\times$ 0·14 = King Armstrong (KA) U/l KA U/l $\times$ 7·1 = i.u./l
Glutamate pyruvate transaminase (SGPT)	i.u./l = mU/ml
Creatine phosphokinase (CPK)	No conversion necessary
Amylase	i.u./1 $\times$ 0·54 = Somogyi U/l Somogyi U/l $\times$ 1·85 = i.u./l
Sodium, potassium, chloride (equivalent weights Na 23 g, K 39 g, Cl 35·5 g)	mmol/l = mEquiv/l
Calcium (equivalent weight 20 g)	mmol/l $\times$ 4 = mg/100 ml mg/100 ml $\times$ 0·25 = mmol/l mmol/l $\times$ 2 = mEquiv/l

Inorganic phosphorus	$mmol/l \times 3.1 = mg/100\ ml$
(equivalent weight P 31 g)	$mg/100\ ml \times 0.32 = mmol/l$
Plasma cortisols	$\mu g/100\ ml \times 27.6 = nmol/l$

Appendix 1.14. Submission of Samples to the Laboratory

Blood

Biochemistry

Anticoagulants: The majority of blood biochemical estimations can be made on either serum or plasma. If an anticoagulant is used, it is usually heparin: exceptions are in the measurement of glucose where a fluoride (usually in combination with oxalate) anticoagulant is used to prevent glycolysis, and in ammonia estimation where EDTA is used. Calcium estimations must be made using plasma.

Volume: The volume of blood required is obviously dependent on the method of estimation. In general, 1 ml of blood is sufficient for each test, though less may be needed if an autoanalyser is used.

Storage: Biochemical estimations should be carried out as soon as is practicable. If samples have to be sent to another laboratory it is highly preferable to separate the serum or plasma first. Haemolysed samples are unsuitable for colorimetric techniques and potassium and inorganic phosphorus results are falsely elevated from unseparated samples. Samples should be stored at 4 °C until tested or dispatched.

Haematology

Anticoagulant: EDTA (ethylenediamine tetra-acetic acid) (Sequestrene) is the only satisfactory anticoagulant for routine haematology. Haemoglobin concentration can be measured on other samples, e.g. heparin.

Volume: 1 ml of blood is adequate for routine haematology.

Storage: Blood cells deteriorate on storage. If samples have to be stored (this should be at 4 °C) or posted, it may be advisable to make a blood film at the time of collection. This should be air-dried and stored at room temperature. The presence of blood parasites such as haemobartonella can only be demonstrated on such fresh blood smears.

Urine

Urine for analysis, if this is not to be carried out immediately, benefits from the addition of a preservative, e.g. boric acid (Sterilin universal container, Sterilin, Teddington, Middx). Samples preserved with boric acid are also suitable for subsequent bacterial culture.

Faeces

Faeces should always be submitted in air-tight screw-topped containers.

Swabs for bacteriological examination

Swabs taken for bacteriological culture should be placed in suitable transport media, e.g. Stewart's, before despatch to the laboratory. All samples should be sent without delay. Certain examinations, e.g. faeces for campylobacter, may require specialized media or techniques and the appropriate laboratory should be contacted for details.

Material for virological examination

It is advisable to check with the laboratory concerned as to the best method of transport. Some samples, e.g. oropharyngeal swabs, require virus transport media (VTM), which may usually be obtained from the laboratory.

Appendix 2

Histological Fixatives

The most widely used fixative in histopathology is formaldehyde which is commercially available as a solution containing 35–40 per cent gas by weight (40 per cent formaldehyde known as 'formalin').

For tissue fixation formaldehyde is used as a 4 per cent solution giving 10 per cent formalin and is most widely used either as formol saline or neutral buffered formalin solution. The latter solution has the advantage of preventing the formation of formalin pigment which occurs with non-buffered acid formaldehyde solutions.

Formol saline

40% formaldehyde	100 cm^3
Sodium chloride	9 g
Tap-water	900 cm^3

Neutral buffered formalin

40% formaldehyde	100 cm^3
Distilled water	900 cm^3
Sodium dihydrogen phosphate monohydrate	4 g
Disodium hydrogen phosphate (anhydrous)	6·5 g

It cannot be emphasized too strongly that tissues must be fixed in wide-necked bottles so that removal is easy and there is no distortion of the preserved material. There must also be sufficient fixative to completely cover the specimen and allow for quick and adequate penetration.

Appendix 3

UK Regulations on Postal Transmission of Pathological Specimens

The Post Office guide, in the section on packing and make-up, makes the following statements about sending pathological specimens through the post:

Pathological specimens – articles sent for medical examination or analysis

Deleterious liquids or substances, though otherwise prohibited from transmission by post, may be sent for medical examination or analysis to a recognized medical laboratory or institute, or to a qualified medical practitioner or a registered dental practitioner or veterinary surgeon by first class letter post, but on no account by parcel post, under the following conditions:

1. Any such liquid or substance must be enclosed in a receptacle, hermetically sealed or otherwise securely closed, and this receptacle must itself be placed in a strong outer container, e.g. of wood, metal or fibreboard (or other container which has been approved by the Post Office) in such a way that it cannot shift about. In some cases it will be necessary to enclose the receptacle in an emergency containment, e.g. polythene bag, before it is placed in a strong outer container. A sufficient quantity of some absorbent material such as absorbent paper tissues or absorbent cotton wool must be packed about the receptacle as absolutely to prevent any possible leakage from the package in the event of damage to the receptacle. The packet so made up must be conspicuously marked FRAGILE WITH CARE and bear the words PATHOLOGICAL SPECIMEN.

2. Any packet of the kind found in the parcel post, or found in the letter post not packed and marked as directed, will be at once stopped and destroyed with all its wrappings and enclosures. Further, any person who sends by post a deleterious liquid or substance for medical examination or analysis other than as provided by these regulations is liable to prosecution.

3. All forms of packaging for pathological specimens intended for transmission by post must be approved by the Post Office. In all cases a complete specimen pack together with details of the nature and quantities of the contents must be submitted for approval to Postal Headquarters (PMk 1.3) St Martin's-le-Grand, London EC1A 1HQ. Approval is given only in respect of the contents described. Before a pack may be used for any other contents the Post Office must be consulted.

Appendix 4

Pathology Request and Report Forms

Department of Veterinary Pathology, University of Liverpool
Request for Necropsy/Surgical Pathology

Pathology Lab. No.

Clinic accession no.	*Received*
Species *Breed*	*Date of necropsy*
Age *Sex*	*Reported*
Owner	*Tissue(s)*
University clinician	*Interval between* *death and necropsy*
Referring veterinary *surgeon*	*Body weight*
Date & time of *death/euthanasia/surgery*	*Photograph(s)*
Previous Path. Lab. No(s).	

Clinical features (including anatomical site of surgical specimens)

Differential diagnosis/clinical impression

Department of Veterinary Pathology, University of Liverpool
Necropsy Report

Pathology Lab. No. PM79/188

Clinic accession no.   2219/79   *Received*   26.10.79

Species (C) *Breed* Alsatian   *Date of necropsy*   26.10.79

Age 6 months *Sex* M   *Reported*   5.11.79

Owner   Chadwick

University clinician   —   *Interval between*
                                            death and necropsy   2 hrs.
Referring veterinary
   surgeon   —   *Body weight*   11 kg.

Date & time of   10.15   *Photograph(s)* Museum specimen
   ~~death~~*/euthanasia*   26.10.79

Previous Path. Lab. No(s).

Clinical features
   Steatorrhoea, failure to thrive, coprophagia. Negative for faecal trypsin. Fat and
   starch present in faeces.
   Exocrine pancreatic insufficiency.

Histology reference: H 1440-79

EXTERNAL EXAMINATION: A poorly grown emaciated dog with a fresh un-
sutured mid-line laparotomy incision. Conspicuous protrusion of the vertebrae.

SKIN: Subcutaneous tissues contain very little adipose tissue. There is no evidence
of haemorrhage or oedema.

ALIMENTARY SYSTEM: Unremarkable teeth, tongue, mouth, salivary glands and
oesophagus. Normal-sized empty stomach is lined by rugose mucous membrane. The
small intestines are unremarkable. The caecum, colon and rectum are grossly distended by bulky pale rancid faeces. The liver is of normal size and colour with
smooth glistening capsular surfaces and even firm dark cut surfaces. Biliary tract and
gallbladder are lined by normal smooth green mucous membrane and normal fluid
green bile can be expressed easily into the duodenum. The pancreas is uniformly
grossly reduced in size. The tail of the duodenal limb is represented by a few pale
cream areas of mesenteric thickening up to only a few mm in greatest dimension.
Peritoneum is smooth and glistening without excess fluid.

RESPIRATORY SYSTEM: Unremarkable upper respiratory tract. Larynx, trachea
and bronchi are lined by smooth glistening pale mucous membranes. The lungs are
aerated, pink and dry and collapse on opening the chest. Pleura is smooth and glistening without excess fluid.

CARDIOVASCULAR SYSTEM: Unremarkable pericardial sac without excess fluid.

Normal right and left ventricles and atria with firm even dark myocardial cut surfaces. Cardiac valves are smooth, slender, glistening and transparent. Major vessels are unremarkable.

LYMPHORETICULAR TISSUES: Slightly distended spleen with smooth glistening capsular surface and congested dark cut surfaces. Lymph nodes are conspicuous, but not abnormally so for a dog of this age. Tonsils are unremarkable. Bone-marrow is not examined.

URINARY SYSTEM: The capsules strip with ease from the smooth pale cortical surfaces of the even-sized kidneys. On the cut surfaces there is normal cortico-medullary demarcation. Unremarkable pelvis, ureters, bladder and urethra.

GENITAL SYSTEM: Small flabby scrotal testes with smooth tunicae. Cut surfaces of the testis are pale, even and soft. One testis is fixed whole in formalin. Normal juvenile prostate. Unremarkable urethra.

MUSCULOSKELETAL SYSTEM: Skeletal muscle is grossly reduced in bulk but the colour and consistency are unremarkable. Major joints are unremarkable. The bones fracture with normal ease. Nervous system is not examined.

ENDOCRINE SYSTEM: Adrenals and thyroid are unremarkable to casual examination and are fixed whole. Cut surfaces are unremarkable.

MACROSCOPIC DIAGNOSIS

1. Pancreatic degeneration

MICROSCOPIC

PANCREAS: Normal ducts and blood vessels are present but exocrine component is represented only by small lobules of small cells with pale-staining granular cytoplasm. The normal eosinophilic/basophilic cytological differentiation is not present. There is no fibrosis, nor is there any inflammatory component.

SUBMAXILLARY SALIVARY GLAND: No significant abnormality is recognized.

MESENTERIC LYMPH NODE: No significant abnormality is recognized.

TESTES: No sperm are present in epididymis or seminiferous tubules.

DUODENUM: No significant abnormality is recognized. In particular there is no
COLON: evidence of lipofuscin in intestinal smooth muscle.

COMMENT: A case of pancreatic malabsorption in a young dog associated with advanced degeneration of pancreatic acinar tissue.

Appendix 5

Check-list of Organs for Gross Post-mortem Examination (Small Animals)

EXTERNAL EXAMINATION

SKIN, SUBCUTANEOUS TISSUE, FAT, NAVEL

ALIMENTARY SYSTEM: Teeth, tongue, mouth, salivary structures, oesophagus, stomach, intestines, anus and anal sacs, liver, biliary tract and gallbladder, pancreas. Peritoneum, omentum.

RESPIRATORY SYSTEM: Nares, nasal chambers, sinuses, pharynx, larynx, trachea, bronchi, lung, pleura.

CARDIOVASCULAR SYSTEM: Pericardium, ventricles and atria, myocardium, valves, aorta, venae cavae, arteries, veins.

LYMPHORETICULAR TISSUES: Spleen, thymus, lymph nodes, lymphatics, tonsils, bone-marrow.

URINARY SYSTEM: Kidney, ureters, bladder, urethra.

GENITAL SYSTEM: Ovaries, uterus, fetus, placenta, cervix, vagina, vulva, mammary glands. Scrotum, testes, tunica vaginalis, vas deferens, penis, prepuce, prostate.

MUSCULOSKELETAL SYSTEM: Skeletal muscle, diaphragm, joints, bones, spine. Bursae, tendon sheaths.

NERVOUS SYSTEM: Meninges, brain, spinal cord, peripheral nerves, eyes, ears.

ENDOCRINE SYSTEM: Adrenals, thyroid, parathyroid, pituitary.

MICROBIOLOGY

TISSUES FOR HISTOLOGY

MACROSCOPIC DIAGNOSIS

MICROSCOPIC

Index